SURGICAL SCRIPTS

Master Surgeons
Think Aloud About
43 Common Surgical Problems

Charles M. Abernathy, MD
Professor of Surgery
University of Colorado School of Medicine
Denver, Colorado

Robert M. Hamm, PhD
Director, Program in Clinical Decision Making
Department of Family Medicine
University of Oklahoma College of Medicine
Oklahoma City, Oklahoma

HANLEY & BELFUS, INC./ Philadelphia
MOSBY/ St. Louis • Baltimore • Boston • Chicago • London
Philadelphia •Sydney • Toronto

Publisher: HANLEY & BELFUS, INC.
               210 S. 13th Street
               Philadelphia, PA 19107
               (215) 546-7293
               FAX (215) 790-9330

North American and worldwide sales and distribution:

               MOSBY
               11830 Westline Industrial Drive
               St. Louis, MO 63146

In Canada: Times Mirror Professional Publishing, Ltd.
               130 Flaska Drive
               Markham, Ontario L6G 1B8
               Canada

Library of Congress Cataloging-in-Publication Data

Surgical scripts : master surgeons think aloud about 43 common surgical problems /
Charles M. Abernathy, Robert M. Hamm.
       p.   cm.
    Includes index.
    ISBN 1-56053-119-3 (soft)
    1. Surgery—Decision making—Case studies.   1. Hamm, Robert M., 1950–
    |DNLM: 1. Surgery—case studies.   2. Decision Making—case studies.
    WO 16 A146s 1994|
    RD31.5.S88   1994
    617—dc20
    DNLM/DLC
    for Library of Congress   93-39297
                                                                       CIP

SURGICAL SCRIPTS   ISBN 1-56053-119-3

Library of Congress catalog card number   93-39297

Last digit is the print number: 9   8   7   6   5   4   3   2   1

In Memoriam

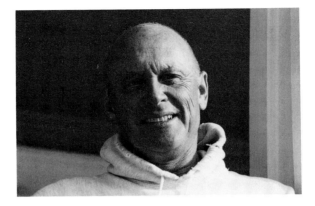

CHARLES M. ABERNATHY, M.D.

1941–1994

Author & Friend

It is with profound sorrow that we report the death on March 24, 1994 of the first author, Dr. Charles M. Abernathy, the very day that this book was scheduled to go to press. This page cannot adequately capture him—his life, his work, his personal and professional accomplishments—or everything he meant to those of us privileged to have known him. Charlie (he would have insisted that formality stop here) was not only the first author of Hanley & Belfus but our unequaled friend and staunchest supporter. His earlier book with us, called *Surgical Secrets*, became an acclaimed best-seller and the forerunner of "The Secrets Series," which Charlie edited.

Charlie was a man of the American West. We suspect he would have preferred to be remembered as a simple country surgeon. Yet his down-to-earth style masked an intensely scientific mind, which kept him in constant search for better answers to problems in medical education, biomedical science, and clinical practice.

He was also an incisive, decisive man of action. Charlie exuded a force. He made things happen; he got the job done. He knew what was important. His forward vision and prolific creativity broke barriers and expanded the horizons of our company. He challenged and inspired us to accomplish more than we ever would have without him. And he made it fun.

We gratefully acknowledge that he made a lasting contribution to the style and quality of our publications. We sincerely believe that this new book, *Surgical Scripts*, and its forthcoming companion, *Surgical Intuition*, will represent his finest contributions to the surgical world that he served with piercing insight and passion.

Linda Belfus
Publisher

CONTENTS

PART I: MASTER SURGEON THINK-ALOUDS

1.   Melanoma   **3**

2.   Carotid Endarterectomy Subsequent to Stroke   **7**

3.   Unconscious Football Player   **15**

4.   Victim of Motor Vehicle Accident
        with Dilated and Sluggish Pupils   **19**

5.   Breast Mass   **23**

6.   0.5-cm Breast Cancer   **27**

7.   Vague Breast Mass   **29**

8.   Large Breast Mass   **35**

9.   Stab Wound to Chest   **39**

10.   Thoracic Outlet Syndrome   **43**

11.   Liver Metastases   **45**

12.   Cancer of Pancreas   **49**

13.   Mass in Pancreas   **55**

14.   Postcholecystectomy Duct Injury   **59**

15.   Melena   **61**

16.   Adenocarcinoma of Stomach   **63**

17.   Gastric Ulcer   **67**

18.   Gastric Outlet Obstruction   **71**

19.   Small Bowel Obstruction with Hypoxic Episode   **75**

20.   Bleeding Duodenal Ulcer   **81**

21.   Right Lower Quadrant Pain   **85**

22.   Pelvic Fracture   **89**

23.   Villous Adenoma of Rectum   **93**

24.   Rectal Cancer   **95**

Contents

PART II: EXPERT/NOVICE THINK-ALOUDS

25.   Campfire Burn   **104**

26.   Burn in Apartment Fire   **108**

27.   Acute Carotid Dissection   **112**

28.   Cerebral Vascular Accident   **116**

29.   Thyroid Nodule   **120**

30.   Pacemaker Complication   **124**

31.   Solitary Pulmonary Nodule   **128**

32.   Sepsis of Unknown Focus   **136**

33.   Liver Laceration from Motor Vehicle Accident   **140**

34.   Hemorrhagic Pancreatitis   **146**

35.   Laparoscopic Cholecystectomy   **148**

36.   Jaundice with Pain   **152**

37.   Epigastric Pain   **158**

38.   Abdominal Aortic Aneurysm   **162**

39.   Left Lower Quadrant Pain   **166**

40.   Small Bowel Obstruction   **170**

41.   Pelvic Fracture   **174**

42.   Rectal Bleeding   **180**

43.   Acute Pain in Leg   **186**

Index   **191**

CONTRIBUTORS

The authors gratefully acknowledge the following individuals for their time and assistance in participating in the think-alouds in this book:

Craig Anderson	Ed Hartford	Denise Norton
Tom Beaver	Gilbert Hermann	Jim Pareso
Denis Bensard	Whit Hollis	Nate Pearlman
Walt Biffl	Scott Hurlbert	Brad Pickhardt
Betsy Brew	Rick Kline	Jack Pickleman
Ramon Buerger	Bill Krupski	Dimitri Pyrros
Brad Bute	Ham Lokey	Bob Read
Jeff Clark	John Lung	Tom Rehring
Joe Cleveland	Robert MacDonald	Christine Rogness
Jeff Cross	Phil Mallory	Randy Ross
Steve Danahey	Bob McCurdy	Robert Rowland
Debbie Davis	Rob McIntyre	Bob Rutherford
Mike Disney	Steve Milheim	Robert Schreiber
Ben Dykstra	Mary Mockus	John Sharp
Tina Finlayson	Fred Moore	John Simon
Reg Franciose	Gene Moore	John Sun
Jack Gallagher	Joyce Moore	Tom Takach
Sharon Hammond	John Nichols	Bruce Waring
Alden Harken	Mark Nishaya	Rebecca Wiebe

Acknowledgment: Our sincere appreciation to Yvonne Taylor for her work in transcribing the scripts and preparing the manuscript.

FOREWORD

It is reasonable to believe if we know how we learn, we will do better at learning. For two thousand years this has been a challenge. In this book and its companion volume, *Surgical Intuition*, Drs. Abernathy and Hamm focus on how surgeons make time-constrained decisions concerning complex clinical problems. They champion surgeons' intuition, the use of judgment based on experience to select pre-programmed solutions that are instantly available through pattern recognition. This contrasts with the more laborious hypothetico-deductive reasoning, in which a clinician hypothesizes *a priori* a diagnosis on the basis of data obtained from a history and physical examination, then perhaps chooses a test to confirm or deny the hypothesis, and on the basis of the result either further tests the hypothesis or discards it and switches to another hypothesis. Hypothetico-deductive reasoning becomes complicated whenever multiple, often conflicting factors must be considered. The team of an experienced clinical surgeon and an equally trained cognitive psychologist makes a strong case for pattern recognition when conflicting forces on decision synthesis cause mental gridlock. In *Surgical Intuition*, they establish the foundation for their thesis. In this volume, *Surgical Scripts*, they apply the thesis to case studies. This book therefore both supports the scientific basis for their learning-logic and provides students (of all ages) practical suggestions of how to achieve clinical wisdom in complex clinical problem solving. By analyzing the difference between problem-solving methods of junior residents and acknowledged experts, they identify how the novice can more efficiently reach the pattern recognition that characterizes the thought processes of master surgeons.

As one who has spent more than a decade exploring and advocating use of hypothetico-deductive reasoning in surgical teaching, how do I evaluate this contrarian approach advocated by my cherished colleague, Dr. Abernathy, who since his early resident days has consistently been an iconoclast—much to our mutual delight and profit? I resolve our differences by a suggested compromise, which Abernathy will predictably interpret as weakness! I suggest that algorithms and the logic process using Bayesian theory to revise one's prior probabilities are the ways we solve most simple clinical problems, while some variation of pattern recognition is the intuitive approach we turn to when information overload causes mental gridlock in seeking an answer. Wherever "truth" lies in seeking ways to understand how clinicians arrive at logical conclusions in patient management, the search will inevitably improve our methods of teaching and ultimately result in better decision making.

The case studies in this book are analogous to those used for half a century in law and business schools. With the help of the analysis of the decision making process in each scenario in this book, surgical residents and all clinical surgeons should improve their efficiency in solving clinical problems—the goal of every physician.

Ben Eiseman, M.D.
Emeritus Professor of Surgery
University of Colorado Health Sciences Center
Veterans Affairs Distinguished Physician
Denver, Colorado

PREFACE

The Heisenberg Uncertainty Principle says the more accurately you know the position of the object, the less certain you are of where it is going—its momentum. Conversely, if you know the momentum very accurately, then you can't be quite sure where it is. This is also true in clinical surgery: The more you have to concentrate on knowing precisely the state of the disease process at a given moment, the less likely you are to try to project what direction the process is going to take in the future. The intuitive processes of surgery are typically involved more in figuring out what is going to happen in the future, and less with what is the case at the present moment. Just as theoretical physicists use "thought experiments," surgeons can use "scripts" about patients to teach the thought processes.

Contained in the surgical scripts are the relevant questions. As the experts' thoughts flow from one concept to another, questions come to mind that the surgeon knows he or she can answer by using available data or by observing changes in the patient's course. These are the questions that both make a difference and can be answered.

The following 43 surgical scripts are actual thinking aloud by surgeons, lightly edited. The first section is by master surgeons alone. The second section shows the thoughts of expert and novice surgeons in parallel so the reader may compare and contrast them. To help you find scripts about particular problems, the think-alouds are presented "outside in" and "top down" within the master surgeon and expert/novice sections.

The surgeons were presented with "paper patients" and were given relatively little specific clinical information. The case descriptions presented here contain much less detail than the cases that appear in the Clinical Problem Solving feature of the *New England Journal of Medicine*, in an attempt to discover surgeons' basic scripts as they respond about a particular patient. We feel that inclusion of less detail in these scenarios allows the issues considered most important by the surgeon to "bubble up." The surgeon must make assumptions to fill in the gaps and then take the problem from there. Two surgeons may be talking about different patients, and their responses, therefore, may diverge appropriately, revealing two alternative scripts pertinent to the case.

Some of the think-alouds are different from how the surgeon would talk when faced with a real case, where talking may be inhibited by thoughts such as, "Quick, what do you do?" and "Don't waste your listeners' time with unnecessary process details." The master surgeons were often relaxed, stepping through the whole script at one sitting, using the default values (most common appearance), with attention to the dangers— other hypotheses, whether common or uncommon—that present risks that need to be taken account of.

Typical instructions to the surgeon were:
"I'll turn on the tape recorder. I'll present the case and you tell me your thoughts. You can ask for information. I may or may not respond to that request. And then I'll give you some more data at a later point, as we go through the case."

The cases in the expert/novice think-alouds were presented in a group context. While the rest of the residents ate their pizza, the participants stepped out of the room and then came back in, one at a time, from junior to senior, to give their response to the same script.

Following each think-aloud, Abernathy presents observations from the surgeon's perspective and Hamm presents a commentary from the cognitive psychologist's perspective.

The think-alouds are intended to underscore the relation between ideas and behavior as expert knowledge develops. The resident is in the process of developing the intellectual framework for considering all sides of the issues specific to a problem. With several more years of experience, the resident's behavior is likely to catch up with his or her ideas. This shows the importance of talking surgical philosophy, of hashing out the issues during residency. Such discussions may not have an immediate influence on residents' behavior, but they lay the groundwork for the appropriate decisions later.

The surgeons' and residents' responses to the problems presented in all 43 think-alouds in this book illustrate how to solve diagnostic and therapeutic problems—how to search for solutions. Surgeons' knowledge, contained in scripts such as those illustrated in this book, lets them find what they know quickly—and this in turn speeds up their search for the answer to the patient's problem.

We hope that experts and novices alike will find the scripts presented here both challenging and instructive.

Charles M. Abernathy, M.D.
Robert M. Hamm, Ph.D.

PART I

MASTER SURGEON THINK-ALOUDS

Throughout the master surgeon think-alouds, **boldface type** is used to signify the voice of the presenter (one of the authors) of the case. The master surgeons' responses are in regular typeface and indented. The Surgical Observations are boxed and numbered to correlate with statements made by the master surgeon. The Surgical Observations, written by Dr. Abernathy, are intended to explain or characterize the master surgeon's thoughts about a particular facet of the case. The Cognitive Psychologist's Commentary, written by Dr. Hamm, addresses a key feature of the think-aloud that is summarized in a boldfaced statement and then discussed in more detail.

1. Melanoma
2. Carotid Endarterectomy Subsequent to Stroke
3. Unconscious Football Player
4. Victim of Motor Vehicle Accident with Dilated and Sluggish Pupils
5. Breast Mass
6. 0.5-cm Breast Cancer
7. Vague Breast Mass
8. Large Breast Mass
9. Stab Wound to Chest
10. Thoracic Outlet Syndrome
11. Liver Metastases
12. Cancer of Pancreas
13. Mass in Pancreas
14. Postcholecystectomy Duct Injury
15. Melena
16. Adenocarcinoma of Stomach
17. Gastric Ulcer
18. Gastric Outlet Obstruction
19. Small Bowel Obstruction with Hypoxic Episode
20. Bleeding Duodenal Ulcer
21. Right Lower Quadrant Pain
22. Pelvic Fracture
23. Villous Adenoma of Rectum
24. Rectal Cancer

1. MELANOMA

A 28-year-old man is referred to you by an internist. The patient has a 0.3-cm pigmented lesion of the left scapular area. You obtain a biopsy. The pathologist designates it a Clark's level II Breslow 0.92 mm lesion. The patient has no palpable nodes. What are your thoughts?

This patient has a very favorable prognosis and I try to convey that to him during the course of my evaluation. ☐ I also try to ascertain whether he has any masses or similar problems, and whether there is any family history or clinical history of the dysplastic nevus syndrome in order to determine how carefully he needs to be followed and how carefully the rest of his skin needs to be scrutinized.

Usually when I receive referrals of such patients from dermatologists, they have had some kind of punch biopsy, although dermatologists are becoming more aggressive in doing the needle biopsy. Then they refer patients to me when the pathologist says the tumor is close to, less than a millimeter from, the surgical margin. Then I explain exactly what needs to be done to try to assure the patient that the disease will not come back in the region, and I tell them why—because it has been well shown that if a melanoma recurs, the outlook is very poor for most patients who have recurrent melanoma at the primary site. Then we talk about what additional things might be considered. For a scapular lesion, of course, the lymph drainage areas are multiple. ☐

For a stage I lesion with no palpable axillary or cervical lymph nodes, it is my bias that patients do best when followed without doing so-called prophylactic lymph-adenectomies. I schedule the patient for surgery, usually under local anesthesia, and I re-excise the lesion, trying to obtain 1-cm margins in all directions, including the fat down to the fascia of the musculature of the scapula. I personally see the patient 3 or 4 times a year for the first 4 years, checking the site of involvement, the regional lymph nodes, and the rest of the skin. Although some patients do not return (some of them end up going back to the dermatologist), I recommend that they do. ☐

The patient returns in about 9 months and has what to you feels like a palpable lymph node in the left posterior neck over the trapezius muscle.

At that point he needs a thorough search for additional disease to see where he's moved from stage II to stage III disease. He needs a chest x-ray, a complete physical evaluation, baseline blood studies, and chemistry profile primarily. ☐ Then I tell the patient that the lesion is going to have to be biopsied and that this needs to be done in surgery. In surgery I make an incision that allows me to resect those lympathics in the posterior part of the neck, which is a difficult area in which to obtain a good clean lymphadenectomy. It is just not an area where there is a lot of lymphatic tissue, especially in an obese patient, so you end up getting 3 or 4 lymph nodes, including the involved node. I don't think there is anything to offer this patient, aside from doing an extensive radical lymphadenectomy.

Okay. You do that and indeed it was one melanoma node. None of the other tests showed any problem at all. You continue to follow the patient and he returns in 6 months. This time he has little black dots about 3 cm in a circle around the previous incision over his left scapular area.

I'd tell him it's a good idea at this point if he goes on a cruise.

Surgical Observations

[1] The surgeon begins with the thought that overall the patient is going to have a very favorable prognosis. It is the first statement that he makes.

[2] As he is talking to the patient, the surgeon is also thinking about technical considerations such as the multiple areas that this lesion could drain to. Surgeons frequently find themselves thinking through the problem as they are discussing it with the patient. Sometimes the thoughts are vocalized to the patient and sometimes the spoken thoughts are not as technical as the thoughts proceeding in a parallel fashion in the surgeon's mind.

[3] This surgeon has devised a follow-up schedule. Such schedules are difficult to find for specific lesions in the surgical literature, or if they are found, are frequently not specific enough to be applied to the individual case. The surgeon emphasizes he would like to see the patient personally.

[4] Notice that at the time of the recurrence, the surgeon *first mentions* the need for chest and laboratory evaluation. He has used the knowledge that the laboratory and x-ray evaluation in the initial presentation of the patient would have been of low yield and no real value, and goes only to the "staging" of the patient at this time.

Expert surgeons' thoughts are organized as if they are talking to patients.

Cognitive Psychologist's Commentary: Melanoma

An expert surgeon's knowledge is organized efficiently and pragmatically. The efficient organization accounts for the surgeon's ability to access rapidly any parts of a large body of knowledge. Someone may have knowledge "in there," but if it is not organized to be quickly accessible when needed, it is of little practical use.

Knowledge does not become rapidly accessible through efficient study of organized facts in textbooks. Rather, the efficient knowledge organization is developed through repeated experience.[1] It is made both complicated and accessible by being used again and again in situations with only slight variations. This fact makes organization of knowledge "pragmatic," that is, the knowledge is organized around the situations in which it is typically used.

The pragmatic nature of expert knowledge can be seen in this transcript. The surgeon thinks about a case as if talking with the patient. Thoughts relevant to diagnosis (family history, presence of masses, biopsy options), the treatment decision (excision without prophylactic lymphadenectomy), and prognosis (recurrence of melanoma signals a poor outlook) are expressed in the context of an imagined conversation with the patient.

The expert surgeon, of course, does not need to pretend to be talking with a patient in order to access knowledge pertinent to the diagnosis and treatment of melanoma. Surgeons who teach may also have easy access to facts organized in a "lecture" format. And surgeons who regularly use the knowledge only when dealing with patients can also access it in response to a colleague's question, a board-qualifying exam, or even a crossword puzzle.

The memory in which the surgeon's knowledge is stored can be conceived as a network of ideas; every idea is connected to a number of others that are related or associated in various ways.[2] In such a memory network many paths may lead to an idea. But the paths that are used most frequently are stronger and can retrieve their targets more rapidly. For this reason, the expert surgeon, asked to "think aloud," talks about the patient along with the disease—the surgeon's most frequent access to knowledge occurs when he or she is with patients.

Most of an expert surgeon's thinking about a patient with a routine problem occurs when the surgeon is actually with the patient. When he or she first hears the description of the patient's symptoms, a judgment of the problem and the appropriate treatment forms almost immediately. When meeting with the patient, the surgeon uses the history and physical exam to check and modify the diagnosis and treatment. Of course, test results may trigger changes in plan when the patient is not there. The point is that the surgeon does not set aside 15 minutes to review the facts about each patient and make a decision. Instead, the diagnosis is determined and the treatment decision made while the patient is present. (This is not to say that all pertinent thoughts are expressed to the patient, for the justifications are presented in a well-rehearsed summary statement.) The patient is there, of course, during the surgery, but is not conversing with the surgeon. Thus our surgeon's description of the operation makes no reference to conversation with the patient.

In sum, the surgeon's knowledge of melanoma is organized for easy access in a way that fits with the situation in which it is most frequently used. Because the surgeon does much of the diagnostic thinking and decision making about melanoma patients when talking with patients, when "thinking aloud" about a case description he or she refers spontaneously to what would be said in the conversation with the patient.

1. Patel VL, Evans DA, Kaufman DR: A cognitive framework for doctor-patient interaction. In Evans DA, Patel VL (eds): Cognitive Science in Medicine: Biomedical Modeling. Cambridge, MA, MIT Press, 1989, pp 263–308.
2. Collins AM, Loftus EF: A spreading activation theory of semantic processing. Psychol Rev 82:407–428, 1975.

2. CAROTID ENDARTERECTOMY SUBSEQUENT TO STROKE

A 72-year-old woman with a recent stroke had resultant right hemiparesis that slowly improved over 2 days. Her CT scan shows a 2-cm diameter left hemispheric enhancing lesion. You have been called as a vascular surgeon to consult on the case. What would you do?

The first thing I would do is obtain a duplex scan of the neck and look for a source. Based on the CT scan, one could rule out hemorrhage. Hemorrhage would not enhance on CT. Therefore one can presume that emboli are involved. Emboli are the most common cause of stroke, statistically. The most common source for an embolus would be the extracranial carotid arteries. So a duplex scan would be high on the list of priorities.

Of course you would also want to be sure that the second most common source of an embolus, the heart, is not a potential source. Most of that information could be ascertained by the history—does the patient have known arrhythmias? are there any abnormalities on EKG? and so on. In the absence of any of these problems, I would proceed with a duplex as the next appropriate test.

The Doppler shows right-sided occlusion and a deep left-sided plaque with 70% occlusion. Where would you go from there?

This is not a critical stenosis on the ipsilateral side. We are talking now about a left hemispheric stroke with right hemiparesis. In this situation, one is not forced to think about an emergent or urgent operation. The damage essentially has been done; the patient has had her infarct. And it was a major infarct, based upon a total hemiparesis—not just a little hand that went out. In this instance, I would try not to operate emergently, allowing the lesion to heal and thereby making the operation safer. The fear is that if you operate on an acute infarct you will increase the local edema and "turn a white infarct red." Because of the edema, there is a greater chance of hemorrhage and a greater chance of making the patient worse. Jack Riley showed back in the early 1970s that operating on such patients carries a 60% mortality rate. This is the kind of patient you can maintain on aspirin and anticoagulation, repeating the CT scan with enhancement in another 6–8 weeks and considering operative repair at that time.

You get 6–8 weeks down the line, and you have advised the patient to have what operation? We would like you to visualize how you would do that operation and describe technically how you would do it.

First, in addition to the duplex information, I want confirmation of the data with an arteriogram. Personally, I don't operate on duplex findings alone. Duplex can be misleading and doesn't give you nearly as much information, particularly with respect to what is going on intracranially, as an arteriogram. At the 6–8-week juncture, presuming that the lesion had healed and enhancement had stopped, I would obtain an arteriogram, which I presume would show a similar finding as the duplex scan. Then I would recommend an operation, after informed consent; this situation probably involves a higher stroke rate than the usual 2 or 3% because the patient has an occlusion on the contralateral side. And we know from all the theories that an occlusion on the contralateral side increases the risk of stroke and subsequent complications. Because of that I'd quote a somewhat higher stroke complication rate, perhaps in the range of 5–10% as opposed to 2–3%.

Having accepted this risk and the other risks attendant with the operation, you proceed with surgery.

I would do the surgery with the patient under general anesthesia. Particularly because I teach residents to do this operation, I find it much easier in a teaching situation to use general anesthesia. The operation certainly could be done safely under local anesthesia, which is attractive because one can talk to the patient during the operation, have the patient squeeze a rubber ducky in the right hand to be sure that motor function remains, and so on. But from a teaching standpoint, I find it difficult to do the surgery under local cervical block.

Now tell us exactly how you would do this operation.

With the patient in the proper position—head turned to the opposite side and slightly raised (to decrease bleeding), back elevated with a roll—the neck is prepped and draped. I use a longitudinal incision on the anterior border of the sternocleidomastoid, carry it down through the platysma muscle, onto the anterior border of the sternocleidomastoid muscle, until I see the muscle itself, and retract the muscle laterally until the internal jugular vein is revealed. I dissect the internal jugular vein on the anterior surface and up and down along the entire length of the wound until the facial vein is identified. Then I suture-ligate the facial vein, beneath which is the bifurcation of the common carotid artery.

The next step is to dissect the arterial structures out—by "dissecting the patient away from the arteries," as I like to say it. ⬜ You don't wrench up on the artery and risk dislodging emboli. Instead, you think of it as dissecting the patient away from the artery, leaving the artery intact. Next you isolate the common carotid artery and encircle it with a vessel loop, then repeat the procedure with the external carotid artery and finally the more distal internal carotid artery, which is well away from the lesion. Of course, all neurologic structures are preserved, including particularly the vagus, which gives the recurrent laryngeal, and the hypoglossal, which is located in the top of the wound. You tell the assistant not to pull too hard on the retractor and risk injury to the marginal mandibular nerve, as it courses upward beneath the mandible.

How do you get into the artery, and what do you do from there?

At that point you give the patient systemic heparinization and place clamps on first the internal, then the external common carotid artery, because you don't want to dislodge any emboli. The patient has no less than two indications for a shunt: (1) a recent stroke, ipsilateral to the side you're operating on, is an absolute indication for a shunt, because the tissue is at risk for ischemia and you don't want to rely on collateral flow to maintain perfusion, and (2) the patient has a contra-lateral occlusion, which, as we said earlier, involves much greater risk for stroke. We clearly are going to put a shunt in this patient.

How do you put in this shunt?

You perform the arteriotomy. Don't rush this ☑ because if you rush you may make the arteriotomy in the wrong place or cut the posterior wall of the vessel. You have perhaps 3, 4, 5 minutes to put in the shunt. Take your time.

After the clamps are placed, you make the arteriotomy on the posterolateral aspect of the carotid. Do not make it directly on this anterior aspect; if you do, when you sew it up, the artery will foreshorten. On the other hand, a lateral arteriotomy acts as a spine to hold the artery in its normal anatomic position without foreshortening. This is hard to show except in the operating room, but a posterolateral arteriotomy is made well up into the normal artery. When you can see the glistening endothelium or intima, you know you're well above the lesion.

I use a Pruitt-Inahara shunt, but the choice of shunt is up to the surgeon. I like the Pruitt-Inahara because it has a side point that you can check periodically to be sure that the shunt is patent. You must be careful to do the Pruitt-Inahara shunt under direct vision and not dig into the intima. Digging into the intima allows a potential embolus to reside in the distal end of the shunt, and when you restore flow, the embolus will go straight into the brain. The next step is to inflate gently the balloon of the distal Pruitt-Inahara shunt and to allow back bleeding. Then, once again under direct vision, the assistant removes the clamp on the common carotid artery while you maintain a partial occlusion with your finger to retard bleeding. Then you put in the proximal end of the shunt, having the assistant inflate the balloon to a proper level. Finally, you check the flow by the third port of the Pruitt-Inahara—and you're done.

The description takes longer than placing the shunt.

And now the endarterectomy.

The endarterectomy is the part of the procedure that involves a little bit of art. There is a true knack to finding the right plane. This is why you need practice and why some people feel uncomfortable doing endarterectomies. The temptation is to stay too superficial, ☑ that is, toward the intimal level of the artery. If you do, you will leave a yellow layer behind and surely increase the risk of both restenosis and continued atherosclerosis. You must get beyond that yellow layer. On the other hand, if you go too deep, you enter the adventitia, and then you have a paper-thin covering of the artery that tends to become aneurysmal over time. The goal is to get into a juncture between the outer one-third and the inner two-thirds of the vessel, in the deep part of the media, which is a nice pink—not the darker red of the adventitia, not the yellow of the intima, but a perfect pink. And having reached this layer, you go all the way around in the common carotid artery, cut the lesion in two, and then enter the external carotid to complete your external carotid endarterectomy.

The very last part of the procedure is to find the internal carotid endpoint. Getting the proper endpoint is crucial. You want to feather the endpoint by holding the plaque up toward the patient's brain. Do not hold it down toward the feet because it tends to snap off, and then you have a distal ledge. You want to feather off where the intima changes from diseased to normal by holding the lesion toward the patient's head and teasing it away.

Then you have to close that endarterectomy?

Right. And this is a point of some controversy in vascular surgery—whether or not to close it with a patch. Surgeons who favor a patch think that it decreases the rate of restenosis, and intuitively it seems that it should. But in fact it's hard to prove that in every patient a patch decreases the rate of restenosis.

So what do you do?

I usually close a first-time endarterectomy primarily, if the artery is of normal caliber and the patient of normal size. I patch selectively. If artery is very small, as is frequently the case in small elderly women, then I patch. In patients undergoing reoperation, restenosis has already occurred, and on the second or third time around, I always patch over the vessel. I close a normal-size, first-time carotid endarterectoimy with tiny, millimeter bites.

What do you do in trauma?

It depends on where the injury is and how it can be repaired.

Many times the vessels are shot in two, and you don't have the luxury of patching just one side. Then you're faced with how to bridge the gap. It's always tempting to free up artery and do a primary repair, end to end. Patients with traumatic injury are often young people who have so much elastic in the wall of the artery that it stenoses down if you try to bridge too long of a gap. If you've got to err, in my opinion, err on the side of putting in a vein graft for trauma..

Back to the carotid endarterectomy. Three hours after surgery the patient awakens in the recovery room. The staff notice that over the last 15 minutes the right hemiparesis that previously had improved has become much more dense and the patient's speech has begun to slur. What would you do?

Fortunately we don't face that question often, but it's not uncommon for patients to replay the neurologic episode after having a stroke. The fact that the patient woke up normal and replayed the deficit 3 hours later makes you more nervous than if the patient had replayed the episode on awakening. There are a bunch of algorithms to follow in this situation. Some experts call for an emergency CT scan, some for an emergency duplex scan, some for an emergency arteriogram.

In every hospital I have ever worked in, including the current one, such procedures, in my opinion, are too time-consuming. By the time you get the duplex scan or CT or whatever, precious time has been lost and brain tissue is dying. The one thing that you can do in this situation is to find some technical defect that you missed at the time of operation. Hopefully, you try to avoid this problem by getting a duplex scan or an arteriogram after the endarterectomy, but there may be a technical defect nevertheless. ④

Do you always get an arteriogram?

No. I prefer an intraoperative duplex scan. We are in the process of getting a new machine and training lab technicians.

So what are you going to do with this patient?

We're going to take her back to the operating room. I think it's most expeditious to open the neck again and see if there is anything that we can correct.

Surgical Observations

① In this discussion, we find the surgeon using colorful language to describe the most important features of what he is saying. When he says "dissect the patient away from the arteries," it has so much more meaning to the listener or reader than "very careful dissection while grasping the artery."

② The surgeon emphasizes "don't rush this," as so many vascular surgeons have emphasized to residents during this operation for years. Because the natural tendency is to be somewhat anxious, he makes the "don't rush" thought paramount in his mind both at the time he does the operation and at the time he talks about it in this think-aloud.

③ The surgeon realizes that staying superficial is tempting because it keeps him out of trouble, but he has firmly in his mind that he is not going to be tempted by that.

④ Classic forward thinking is demonstrated by a surgeon who has thought about all of the possibilities both in the literature and from experience on how one might proceed with this complication. He has boiled it down to simply returning to the OR.

The master surgeon anchors and adjusts the operative risk.

Cognitive Psychologist's Commentary:
Carotid Endarterectomy Subsequent to Stroke

The expert surgeon must respond appropriately to the risks of surgical procedures, knowing the probabilities of serious consequences and undertaking risky procedures only when the circumstances demand it, such as when the risk of no operation is comparable or greater. But it is difficult to know the exact risk for a particular, unique patient.

One strategy is to remember different risks for different classes of patient. For example, the surgeon is cognizant of the research on the probability of success in patching an endarterectomy compared with simply closing it. Surgeons who "favor a patch think that it decreases the rate of restenosis, and intuitively it seems that it should. But in fact it's hard to prove that in every patient a patch decreases the rate of restenosis." He goes on to explain when he closes—first-time carotid operation, normal-caliber artery, normal-sized individual. He patches very small arteries, as in small elderly women. And he patches repeat operations.

The knowledge about the probabilities of success of patching versus not patching is not stored and used in the form of a numerical probability. Rather, it is embodied in the rules of action—in the categories of artery for which each option is chosen.

Some situations demand expression of probabilities. When justifying decisions, as in teaching, mortality and morbidity rounds, or communicating with a patient, probability measures of the risk of a procedure are often heard. Here the expert vascular surgeon said the 72-year-old woman would have a stroke rate "probably higher than the usual 2 or 3% . . . because she has an occlusion on the contralateral side." He knows the numbers for the typical patient—2–3%. And he knows that in her case the probability is higher: "We know from all the theories that an occlusion on the contralateral side increases the risk of stroke and subsequent complications." So he adjusts his estimate: "I'd quote her a somewhat higher stroke complication rate, perhaps in the range of 5–10% as opposed to 2–3%."

This probability adjustment has several interesting features. First, note that he is more uncertain about the adjusted probability, giving a range of 5% (from 5–10%) rather than a range of 1% (from 2–3%). Although the greater range may be more appropriate for the subset of patients (when the sample in any study has a smaller n, the estimate of the mean has greater uncertainty), this probably reflects the surgeon's uncertainty in his adjustment rather than the features of the studies from which he learned the numbers.

Second, in revising the probability for this particular patient, the surgeon has used a strategy called **anchoring and adjustment**—recalling a number that holds for a general class and then adjusting it to the characteristics of the particular individual.[1] Here he recalled the stroke complication rate for carotid endarterectomies in general (2–3%) and adjusted it upward to 5–10% for the patient's particular situation (contralateral occlusion, age, history of stroke).

People often use this strategy (see box below). They anchor on a number that is quickly available and then adjust it. When making estimates for the first time, they may put too much weight on the initial anchor (9 for heads and 2 for tails) and adjust it insufficiently. What were your answers for heads and tails? Unless you recognized that the same numbers were multiplied in both cases, you probably produced a higher estimate for heads. (Other demonstrations have had different people try the two tasks.)

Numerical Estimation Exercise[2]

Take a coin from where you keep your change. Flip it and follow the "heads" or "tails" instructions:[3]

Heads. Take 10 seconds to estimate the product of the numbers in the following list. Write your answer on a piece of scrap paper.

9 8 2 7 3 6 4 5

Now do the exercise for tails.

Tails. Take 10 seconds to estimate the product of the numbers in the following list. Write your answer on a piece of scrap paper.

2 3 9 4 8 5 7 6

Now do the exercise for heads.

Did the surgeon make an error in estimating the stroke complication rate for this patient by adjusting from the general rate? It is hard to say. Let us distinguish errors in *stating a probability* from errors in *practice*. (And of course, it is a hypothetical patient.) If he knows the probability for this class of patient, and the "adjustment" was just a rhetorical device for teaching the distinction, then his "5–10%" may be quite accurate. If he used a mental adjustment process, his anchor was accurate, and the amount he adjusted may have been too little, just right, or too much. Surely someone who has studied an area for years will have the ability to adjust probability estimates more accurately than a college student thinking about unfamiliar material. Finally, even if the estimate is inaccurate, it may have no impact on the doctor's behavior in this particular case, because the choice to operate is given in the script, developed over the years by a number of experts, passed down and modified in response to ongoing research, and tuned by objective review.[4]

A guiding phrase. The expert vascular surgeon and teacher has a phrase concerning the dissection of a sclerotic carotid artery: "Dissect the body away from the artery." The one phrase, in the form of an instruction, captures the careful technique needed to avoid risks of embolism. Such a phrase can be central to a surgical script. Heard from an instructor, it can serve as the core around which this part of the script is constructed. And it can always be present during the execution of the script to keep the surgeon oriented and to edify observing residents.

Visual images. In his teaching the surgeon offers visual markers to guide in the endarterectomy: the plane you want to be in is pink, not dark red (that's the adventitia) and not yellow (that's the intima).[5]

Skip the algorithms. If the patient would show evidence of another stroke 3 hours after the operation, the surgeon would return to the OR, open up her neck immediately, and look for a technical defect. He prefers direct vision to emergency use of the CT scan, duplex scan, or arteriogram, because they are too slow, given the serious damage happening right now. In this judgment, he disagrees with the recommendations of several algorithms that have been offered for handling the situation.

Of course, his recommendations could be made into an algorithm, too. But the point is that in such situations, it is the doctor's judgment—of the seriousness of the risk, the temporal nature of the process, the time demands of the visualization procedures and their potential utility, and finally his own ability to see and respond—that produces the decision to open up the neck immediately.[6] (See observations on the Gastric Ulcer think-aloud, pp 67–68.)

1. Hogarth RM: Judgement and Choice. New York, Wiley, 1980.
2. Answer: The product is the same, 9! (factorial) or 362,880.
3. Modified from a demonstration by Tversky A, Kahneman T: Judgment under uncertainty: Heuristics and biases. Science 185:1124–1131, 1974.
4. Abernathy CM, Hamm RM: Surgical Intuition. Philadelphia, PA, Hanley & Belfus, 1994, chapter 7.
5. Abernathy CM, Hamm RM: Surgical Intuition. Philadelphia, PA, Hanley & Belfus, 1994, chapter 10.
6. Abernathy CM, Hamm RM: Surgical Intuition. Philadelphia, PA, Hanley & Belfus, 1994, chapter 8.

3. UNCONSCIOUS FOOTBALL PLAYER

Who are the medical students here? Just two? You're sitting here thinking, "What am I doing with a bunch of general surgeons and one neurosurgeon?" But the problem is, no matter what field you go into, you're going to need to know some basic neurosurgery.

A 16-year-old football player is rendered unconscious for 30 seconds, then walks to the sidelines. You are in the stands and are called to the sidelines to see him. How would you examine him? What would you do?

I am assuming that the *mechanism* was not a fall while he was running for a pass by himself. That suggests subarachnoid hemorrhage, like a spontaneous bleed into a brain tumor, although such a mechanism is unlikely in a 16-year-old. It's not going to be diffuse axonal injury for two reasons: (1) he got up and walked to the sidelines, and (2) diffuse axonal injury is a big mechanism. ①

So it isn't going to be a diffuse axonal injury, because the mechanism is not right. The mechanism is right for a contusion of the brain, a milder form of which is called a concussion. The chance of a subdural hematoma is very small because (1) the mechanism is not right, and (2) he's too young. The possibility of epidural hematoma is also very small. You need a skull fracture. How many times do you fracture a skull with a helmet on? ② Very seldom. So you're looking probably at a contusion, possibly as minor as a concussion.

How would you manage him?

I'd look at three things: level of consciousness, pupillary exam, and best motor response.

Tell us what that means.

There are four levels of consciousness: alert, lethargic, obtunded, or comatose. Alert is what you and I are. Lethargic takes continuous verbal stimulation to keep him awake. If he falls asleep while you are talking to him, that is a bad sign. If it takes continuous manual stimulation to keep him awake, that is an even worse sign; that is obtundation. Comatose is somebody that you can't arouse to interact with you.

He is awake and alert now.

He is awake and alert. How about his pupillary exam?

It is normal.

How about his best motor exam?

Excellent.

He's running up and down the field?

He can jog up and down the field.

He sits out for at least 5 or 6 minutes. ③ Has his neurologic exam changed?

Unchanged.

Then the question is, "Is he laying down any new information? Does he know what the score is?"

He is a little fuzzy on what happened to him.

Boom—he doesn't go back in.

He doesn't go back in the game? Does he go to the hospital?

If he gets any worse, he goes to the hospital immediately. He should only get better from the moment of impact, not worse. ④

You examine him and you talk to him. He is really fuzzy and doesn't know what is going on. He complains of mild headache. You send him to the hospital. Does he have to have a CT scan?

When he gets to the hospital, has he gotten any worse?

He still has retrograde amnesia and keeps repeating the same question, "What happened to me? What happened to me?" But beyond that he is okay.

In my hospital he would get a CT scan. A rural setting is a different story. Sending an ambulance crew 80 miles an hour down the road puts three people in danger. You have to have a better idea—is he really worse? People are going to get better or worse with their neurologic problem. They are not going to stay the same. If he is getting worse—at first he could tell you that the other team was the Centennial Bulldogs and now he can't—then boom, he goes.

I notice you didn't look in his fundi.

No. That wastes time.

Why? Doesn't it help you?

No. You know what his neurologic exam is. You know exactly how his whole brain is functioning.

You don't need a reflex hammer?

I don't need a reflex hammer. You see how you have to take the situation of your practice into account. I could say that every patient who comes through my door needs a CT scan because I practice at a place where you can get CT scans 24 hours a day. You have got to tailor what you do to your resources, and you have got to consider the risk/benefit ratio of what you do. You can go through your algorithm and say that "every patient who's knocked unconscious needs a CT scan," but if you go to Sterling, Colorado, you don't have the resources and have to take the risk of transporting the patient. It's easy to say "get a CT," but you have to think about the paramedics, about the patient. If they're involved in an 80-mph motor vehicle accident, you've cost 3 lives because you did a probably worthless exam and want to cover your butt.

Surgical Observations

[1] As in most modern trauma management, the first thought is **mechanism**, which lets the surgeon drastically narrow the possibilities.

[2] He narrows the diagnostic possibilities even further by **using his own mental script**—that is, he realizes that the mechanism does not fit the epidural or subdural hematoma script and tells you why. He still would accept either as the diagnosis if the symptoms proved to be most consistent with them, but because they do not fit the script, they are set aside in his initial thoughts.

[3] The master surgeon has a good clinical answer to a good clinical question. He wants 5–6 minutes to go by (not "for a while"), and then he reexamines the patient. Note how much more meaning that has than "serial examination of the patient."

[4] Again, a simple but clear answer—**not** "well, that depends on how he was doing neurologically, some patients, etc., etc."

The expert surgeon recognizes and focuses on key elements of the case.

Cognitive Psychologist's Commentary:
Unconscious Football Player

Expert surgeons' thinking is very powerful for several reasons. In addition to the large body of knowledge, organized for rapid access, and the resulting spare capacity,[1] the expert also knows what is important and can focus on the key elements of the case.[2]

Thus, when initially engaged in pattern recognition, the surgeon knows to pay attention to the mechanism of the injury—a tackle involves more force than a spontaneous bleed into a brain tumor, but less than would produce a diffuse axonal injury. Large numbers of possibilities are eliminated through the use of the one, highly diagnostic cue.

Later, he focuses on any changes in the football player's ability to think. Because the boy can reveal his state of consciousness, any more detailed neurologic exam would be redundant. Any deterioration in his awareness would make the surgeon send him to the hospital, because "he should only get better, not worse." As Dreyfus et al.[3] characterize it, the judgments of what is important at any stage are not conscious but "perceptual": the expert sees only the important cues in the situation.

Eddy and Clanton[4] described how expert clinicians condense a case into manageable form, focusing on one or two pivotal findings. In posing and testing hypotheses that can account for this key finding, they often can account for the whole case. Success with this strategy depends, of course, on being able to judge which of many possible features of the case to focus on.

The neurosurgeon's discussion of how the decision to get a CT scan depends on its availability shows the flexibility that is characteristic of expert reasoning. Although the knowledge is organized in accessible scripts, the scripts are always modified for the circumstances. The expert understands the justification for each of the details in the script and can rethink the routine decisions in the script when the situation presents different risks.[5]

---

1. Abernathy CM, Hamm RM: Surgical Intuition. Philadelphia, PA, 1994, chapters 3 and 4.
2. Abernathy CM, Hamm RM: Surgical Intuition. Philadelphia, PA, 1994, chapter 8.
3. Dreyfus HL, Dreyfus SE, Athanasiou T: Mind over Machine: The Power of Human Intuition and Expertise in the Era of the Computer. New York, The Free Press, 1986.
4. Eddy DM, Clanton CH: The art of diagnosis: Solving the clinicopathological exercise. In Dowie J, Elstein A (eds): Professional Judgment: A Reader in Clinical Decision Making. Cambridge, Cambridge University Press, 1988, pp 200–211.
5. Abernathy CM, Hamm RM: Surgical Intuition. Philadelphia, PA, 1994, chapters 6–8.

4. VICTIM OF MOTOR VEHICLE ACCIDENT WITH DILATED AND SLUGGISH PUPILS

A victim of a high-speed motor vehicle accident is unresponsive to deep pain, with both pupils somewhat dilated and sluggish. The vital signs are blood pressure of 120/80 and pulse of 60. What does your exam consist of? How urgent is the CT scan?

Number one, I am not getting enough information. I obviously want to know if he was ejected or if he hit his head on the steering wheel. ①

We don't have any other information.

How long was he down in the field? That's the kind of information that I want to know. I also am not getting a good exam from what I've been told so far. He's unconscious, but I am told he has mildly dilated pupils that are sluggish. That tells me nothing. It still confuses me. You can say that you don't know because he has cataracts or because he's blown away one eye. You can even tell me that you haven't examined him. Any of these answers would be better than telling me that he has bilateral, slightly dilated pupils that are sluggishly reactive. If you can't say whether the pupils react or not, just don't say it. On the basis of that exam, I would say that he is drunk.

Tell us what your neurologic exam would be when called to the ED to see this patient.

Level of consciousness.

He is unresponsive to deep pain stimulus.

What about his pupils?

Mildly dilated and sluggish.

Again, I would look to find out exactly what that "sluggish" means. If they're reactive, he's got a toxic metabolic problem and not a mass problem. ②

So you would look very carefully to see if they are clinically reactive.

If you have to look at one thing, look at the pupils. With white-matter injury, he could have reactive pupils, but it's more unlikely than likely.

Is unresponsiveness much more likely to be toxic metabolic, even in a high-energy motor vehicle accident?

It's a tough call. You're putting me on the line. The patient not only has diffuse axonal injury, but he is drunk too. Nobody goes out at 2:00 in the morning and drives 80 mph without being drunk. ③ But one of the clinchers is, what's his best motor exam? What's he doing?

He doesn't move a single thing when you stimulate him.

Not a thing?

No. He is breathing spontaneously.

That doesn't make sense.

He is breathing spontaneously, but he doesn't move a thing when you rub on his sternum.

Then he has to have two injuries. He doesn't move a thing—he's got to have a spinal cord injury.

Do you ever see people deep enough that they won't move a thing?

Yes. But they have fixed and dilated pupils. ④

They always go hand in hand?

Always. A flaccid paralysis with reactive pupils is a spinal fracture. But if he is breathing spontaneously, he has to have his diaphragm intact. That puts it at C3, 4, 5—keeps your diaphragm alive.

The diagnostic peritoneal lavage (DPL) done by the general surgeons showed 200,000 red cells per high power field. Vital signs are stable. The surgeons want to do a laparotomy. The man is flaccid and unresponsive, but we don't think he's got a broken neck. You got a film that shows no injury down to C6. He's now doing a little posturing. They're getting ready to intubate and to give him succinyl choline.

He needs to be intubated, but it is questionable whether you need to clear C6–7 in his case or just go ahead and intubate him with in-line traction. Does he have any soft-tissue swelling? You've essentially got a normal neck x-ray? I think with in-line traction you can intubate him without cricothyrotomy.

Okay. You intubate him. Now the general surgeons want to take the patient with his not grossly positive (but micropositive) DPL to the OR. He's posturing. Does he need a CT scan before he goes to the OR?

Yes. My inclination is that whatever is causing his mildly positive DPL is not going to kill him before any potentially reversible neurologic problems. You should feel comfortable enough sending a patient for a 30- or 40-minute CT scan with a DPL of 200,000.

Before you intubate him, why not just pull down on his shoulders and get C7 cleared?

Because if his neck is taped to the bed, you can pull his head off if he has a broken neck at C7. And I'd be much concerned over that if his original exam, when he wasn't posturing, clearly showed some cord injury signs.

You get certain clues. You get a gestalt. You get a feeling. If the patient is neurologically intact, what's the chance that he's going to have an unstable neck?

There are going to be only 1 or 2 such cases in your career. If he's going to fracture his neck in a high-speed accident, he's going to take out his cord. You can't walk down to the ED and say, "We are not going to get a C-spine on any patient who doesn't have cord injury." When you have to make tough decisions, ⑤ you have to go with your gut feeling. So you leave the Philadelphia collar, but you shoot off to the OR very quickly. You say the neck is not cleared, but my index of suspicion that he has some kind of injury is very low. Why? Because he is not paraplegic or quadriplegic.

Surgical Observations

① The surgeon wants to know the mechanism.

② The surgeon has a direct one-to-one response to reactive pupils: reactive pupils = no mass problem. Reactive pupils do not rule out a mass 100% or imply that a mass problem won't occur in the future. But for now there is no mass problem.

③ The surgeon has used all of his knowledge, including "life knowledge" outside of medicine, to realize that this is probably drunkenness plus a neurologic injury. But, as the next sentences show, he has devised a practical way to sort out a practical problem.

④ Here is a heuristic problem involving two pieces of data—if the patient is flaccid and the pupils not dilated, the flaccidity is not from the brain injury. This observation would not be found in a textbook; it has been "derived" by the surgeon.

⑤ There is an implication here that "tough decisions" are different from routine ones, or perhaps have a different algorithm. The multiple other factors in this case (DPL of 200,000; unresponsiveness; need to intubate) impinge at once to make this a "tough decision."

The expert surgeon intuitively recognizes diagnostic patterns in trauma.

Cognitive Psychologist's Commentary:
Victim of Motor Vehicle Accident with Dilated and Sluggish Pupils

Of interest here is the power of the neurologic exam as a tool for diagnosing and managing CNS trauma. The expert neurosurgeon's script is built around it. When instant pattern recognition fails him, as at first when the picture is confusing, he goes to this tool to organize his thoughts. He directs his attention explicitly to the three categories: level of consciousness, pupillary response, and best motor exam.

Simultaneously, however, he is engaged in intuitive pattern recognition, identifying the possibility that the man is drunk and focusing on the implications of the neurologic exam for the competing hypotheses: mass-occupying lesion, alcohol toxicity, and combination of the two.

Another feature of the surgeon's thinking is that he articulates and uses categorical rules, such as "flaccid paralysis with reactive pupils means spinal fracture," even though he knows that there can be rare exceptions. He pushes through to the most likely conclusion, to see if it can hold up to scrutiny, before going back to consider the rare exceptions. Thus his thinking is similar to that described by Mitchell and Beach[1]: the decision maker first determines whether the current situation fits a familiar pattern, and only when it does not fit does he or she engage in the more laborious work of consciously figuring out what should be done.[2]

---

1. Mitchell TR, Beach LR: ". . . Do I love thee? Let me count . . ." Toward an understanding of intuitive and automatic decision making. Organiz Behav Hum Decis Making 47:1–20, 1990. See also Montgomery H: From cognition to action: The search for dominance in decision making. In Montgomery H, Svenson O (eds): Process and Structure in Human Decision Making. New York, Wiley, 1989, pp 23–49.
2. Abernathy CM, Hamm RH: Surgical Intuition. Philadelphia, PA, Hanley & Belfus, 1994, chapters 6 and 7.

5. BREAST MASS

A 42-year-old premenopausal woman with a 4-cm breast mass is referred to you. You evaluate her, do a physical exam, do not feel any axillary nodes. You sit down to counsel her about her options. What do you think about? What are her options? How do you talk to her?

A 4-cm mass is right at the borderline based on a study of segmental mastectomy that showed survival equivalent with that of modified radical mastectomy. You really do not know if you can do a segmental mastectomy on a 4-cm mass. You probably can, but it has never been studied. If she is right on the border, I would say that she can qualify for a segmental mastectomy. I think it is probably a safe option for her, with results probably equivalent to those with modified radical mastectomy. ▯

I would advise her to have lumpectomy, plus radiation therapy and axillary node dissection. I would listen to whatever concerns she has about radiation therapy, but a mass of that size still falls within the guidelines. She probably will have fairly good results with this type of procedure.

Who makes the actual decision—you or the patient?

It depends. The younger the woman, the more frequently the patient makes the decision. The older the woman, the more frequently it is the doctor. Where we practice, many people still want to know, "What do you recommend, doctor?" They are willing to go, by and large, with that recommendation. Most younger women want to know every aspect of the case before they proceed, and many will not accept a decision made by the doctor. They want separate procedures—they do not care how many. They want to know every step of every decision that is made. They will not accept the doctor's recommendation blindly.

Why do you think such a patient would choose a modified radical in this setting?

The patient may have some knowledge (that a layperson might have) of problems with radiation therapy, which is necessary with a segmental mastectomy. It may be a layperson's fear of recurrence, which is a realistic possibility. Possibly 5% of patients have a local recurrence with a segmental mastectomy. Patients want to avoid a local recurrence at all costs. They may be absolutely frightened that a speck of cancer is left and do not want to take the risk. They want everything removed, the offending area ablated completely and immediately.

Let us say that she decides on a breast-conserving approach and the margins of the excisional biopsy you perform are reported as positive. What do you do then?

The patient has two options: (1) mastectomy or (2) reexcision of the biopsy site with lymph node dissection at that time.

Visualize how you do a separate lymph node dissection and describe how you do it.

The dissection is done with a small incision below the hairline between the two axillary folds, anterior and posterior. The incision is carried down to the subcutaneous tissue, leaving a little skin flap on the upper surface, and then to the border of the pectoralis major muscle. At that point, the axilla is entered below the pectoralis major muscle, and the fascia overlying the axillary vein is opened. The lymph-bearing tissue is dissected from the vein inferiorly, and the dissection is carried laterally to the latissimus dorsi muscle. That is the lateral margin. The thoracodorsal nerves and vessels are preserved ordinarily. Some people preserve the intercostal brachiocutaneous nerve, but I routinely sacrifice it.

What caused you to begin breast-conserving surgery? Lectures? Journals?

I heard Dr. Bernard Fisher talk about the results of his National Surgical Adjuvant Breast Project (NSABP) study at a meeting I attend weekly. It was a convincing presentation. I heard it more than once, probably over a 22-year span. I had done some of that type of surgery in the past on a case-by-case basis in patients with what would have been termed years ago, "minimal breast cancer," combining lumpectomy with an axillary dissection (which uniformly gave very poor cosmetic results because one incision goes all the way around the axilla and into the breast). The patient had done well. Of course, that anecdote carries no validity whatsoever, but coupled with huge clinical trials, it was convincing. [2]

Surgical Observations

[1] These sentences show how an expert clinician realizes that a breast mass of 3, 4, or 5 cm is really a very vague thing. Exact size doesn't play much of a role in treating individual patients. Over two or three sentences he gives us the notion that he would be willing to do a breast-conserving treatment on most patients who are in this general size group.

[2] Here the surgeon reveals what factors led him to change his surgical practice from the way he was taught as a resident to the present time, 20 years later. He notes that his use of breast-conserving surgery was initiated by two factors. One was a "convincing" talk, perhaps heard more than once, by a surgeon whom he respected as an investigator. The other was that in the years of his practice he had occasion to individualize patients' treatments, including lumpectomy and variations thereof, and watched one or two of these patients do well. Although he realized that anecdotal evidence was not statistically valid, he coupled that with the results of the large randomized trial. This changed his practice.

The surgeon understands that changes based only on new randomized prospective trials are not necessarily good for the individual patient. Thus, general changes in his or her practice happen through a combination of new studies and experience with many individual patients.

The expert surgeon changes his script on the basis of experience as well as research.

Cognitive Psychologist's Commentary:
Breast Mass

Notable here is the central role that the surgeon's knowledge of research plays in his thoughts about what to do for this patient. The surgeon knows what has been studied: results have been reported for each type of operation applied to each category of breast mass. And he knows the probabilities associated with each treatment for each type of mass; for example, segmental mastectomy plus radiation involves a 5% chance of local recurrence.

The surgeon also knows the costs of the various approaches, in terms of both universal reactions (suffering from operations and from radiation and chemotherapy) and individual reactions (response to loss of breasts, fear of remaining cancer).

The following knowledge is needed for a formal decision analysis[1]: the different disease entities and treatments, the probabilities of recurrence for each treatment when applied to each category of breast disease; and the universal and individual evaluative responses to treatments, outcomes, and uncertainties. The master surgeon considers this knowledge when making routine decisions. Statistics about disease outcome may come to mind with special ease when the surgeon talks with a patient with breast cancer. Women tend to want to discuss the decision at great length, because the decision to undergo treatment is voluntary rather than compelled by disabling pain, as with an acute abdomen syndrome, for example.

If the master surgeon is aware of the decision-relevant information, one may expect him to change his practices routinely, as the weight of evidence favoring one procedure over another shifts. But his account of how he began breast-conserving surgery suggests otherwise.

He had heard the argument for breast-conserving surgery repeatedly from a surgeon he respected, including the results of clinical trials. But his own experience played a major role in his decision, even though it was with only a small number of patients. You might have expected him to say: "The statistics convinced me, and when my experience agreed with the statistics, it made the statistics even more compelling." But in effect he said the opposite: "My experience convinced me, even though I should have doubted it because it was anecdotal; and when the clinical trials agreed with my experience, that gave it a lot of weight."

Even when the master surgeon thinks extensively about the statistics, the practices embedded in the scripts he originally learned are resistant to change. One needs to see with one's own eyes that it works when done with one's own hands. This shows the importance to the surgeon of stories, cases known in detail, as opposed to abstractions.[2,3]

1. Abernathy CM, Hamm RM: Surgical Intuition. Philadelphia, PA, Hanley & Belfus, 1994, chapter 7.
2. Riesbeck CK, Schank RC: Inside Case-based Reasoning. Hillsdale, NJ, Erlbaum, 1989.
3. Abernathy CM, Hamm RM: Surgical Intuition. Philadelphia, PA, Hanley & Belfus, 1994, chapter 4.

6. 0.5-cm BREAST CANCER

How do you counsel a 73-year-old woman with a 0.5-cm infiltrating ductal cancer? What do you think she needs?

She probably needs only an excisional biopsy, plus or minus radiation therapy, plus or minus axillary node dissection. I would base any adjuvant therapy on her receptor studies and flow cytometry. If she is in good shape and looks much younger than her stated age, ☐ I would counsel her to have lumpectomy, radiation therapy, and axillary node dissection, which would give the most information about her condition. With a tumor of that size, the likelihood of a positive node is pretty small, probably around 10%. If she has positive nodes, you are going to treat her with adjuvant chemotherapy, which would be the only reasonable alternative at that point, I believe. If her nodes were negative and flow cytometry showed a low S-phase diploid tumor, I do not think I would treat her at all with adjuvant therapy. If she is in bad shape and looks a little older than her stated age, with various comorbid conditions, I may counsel her to have a lumpectomy and then follow her with clinical examination. I think this approach is justified, knowing that lumpectomy and radiation therapy give you the same survival as lumpectomy in this setting.

In your practice, who makes the decision whether or not a patient receives adjuvant chemotherapy? Do all patients see a medical oncologist?

No, they do not. I try and make some decisions myself. If it is absolutely clear that they do not need to see an oncologist, I do not refer them unless the family wants it. I would say that overall approximately 80% see an oncologist for an opinion. I do not think it is necessary in that many cases and probably leads to a lot of expense. The oncologist is probably inclined to treat.

Surgical Observation

☐ It would be difficult to define the statements "in good shape" and "looks much younger than her stated age" in a randomized study or algorithm, and yet the surgeon uses these concepts to determine his therapy. This is a common element in many of these master surgeon think-alouds.

Patient categories have fuzzy boundaries.

Cognitive Psychologist's Commentary:
0.5 cm-Breast Mass

The master surgeon's thoughts in this case illustrate judgments that are difficult to express in terms of rules applied to categories. The decision whether to treat the small infiltrating ductal cancer with lumpectomy alone or with lumpectomy plus radiation and/or node dissection depends on the elderly patient's general state, which cannot be defined in terms of a series of specific features. Stated generally, the surgeon will do the least invasive treatment if the woman is weak. Judgment of weakness can be influenced by a large number of factors, of which the surgeon mentions a few: comorbid conditions, bad overall shape, and looking the stated age or older.

The "judgment" here is complicated by the lack of empirical studies. It has not been proved with random controlled trials in women of this age that lumpectomy plus radiation is more effective than lumpectomy alone in increasing the long-term survival, although at first glance you would think it would be. Because the efficacy is "unknown," it is easier for the surgeon to recommend the less rigorous treatment for a patient who appears weak. If there had been a study with women of this age, it would be harder for the surgeon to justify taking intangible considerations into account unless they had been included in the scope of the study.

Because there is no vocabulary for communicating this sort of judgment as simply as categories and rules can be communicated, large-scale controlled studies tend to increase the use of rules and decrease the use of judgment by the field as a whole. This is not because the judgments are in principle indescribable—psychologists can make precise mathematical models of both categorical judgments and the judgments that integrate information about multiple dimensions in a noncategorical manner.[1] But it is much easier to communicate verbally the categorical than the noncategorical judgments.

---

1. Abernathy CM, Hamm RM: Surgical Intuition. Philadelphia, PA, Hanley & Belfus, 1994, chapter 8.

7. VAGUE BREAST MASS

You are seeing a 41-year-old woman with a vague mass in the left upper outer quadrant of her breast. She has a negative mammogram, and ultrasound reveals that the mass is noncystic. You are examining her.

My thoughts are that this 41-year-old woman probably has a benign lesion in her breast, most likely a cyst. It is a discrete mass, and so I take a history to determine whether she has had any trouble with her breast in the past and, if so, the nature of the problem. Does she have any nipple discharge? If so, what was the nature of the discharge? Then during the course of examining her, if there is a discrete mass, ① I determine whether it involves the underlying skin. I also determine whether or not the axillary and cervical lymph nodes are involved.

Then I tell her the diagnostic possibilities and review the mammograms to see if I can ascertain any additional information. Usually, if I think the mass is a cyst, I go ahead and aspirate it on the spot. I use a small 30-gauge needle with 1% Xylocaine, then an 18-gauge needle for aspiration. If it's not a cyst, I do a fine-needle aspiration and proceed from that point. If it's a cyst and fluid is not bloody, I reassure the patient there is no reason to forward the fluid for analysis. Patients frequently want to know that. If the fluid is bloody and I feel that the tap was clean and that I didn't introduce the blood, then I usually forward the fluid to cytology. The vast majority of the time, ② the fluid is not bloody, and the mass goes away. I reassure the patient and tell her to come back in 6 weeks to 3 months, depending on her history—for example, whether or not she has had this problem before.

The fine-needle aspirate comes back confirmatory for ductal carcinoma of the breast. The patient is back in your office, and you're talking to her about that diagnosis.

At that point, I sit down with the patient and her family or whomever she wants involved in the decision making and talk about options. I usually lead off with a little bit about the history and treatment of breast cancer. I spend about 20 or 30 minutes with the patient because I think it is very important. We talk about treatment options, basically about breast-conserving therapy vs. mastectomy. I try to explain what each entails. We also briefly discuss breast reconstruction, especially in the 41-year-old patient. And usually we talk about adjuvant chemotherapy. I detail exactly what a mastectomy entails—removal of a portion of the skin as well as the nipple—and why the nipple and axillary lymph nodes are removed.

I also explain in somewhat less detail exactly what radiation therapy entails—6–6½ weeks, Monday through Friday—what the complications are, and the fact that patients usually experience no systemic problems as a consequence of radiotherapy. I usually don't get involved in a long discussion about adjuvant chemotherapy because it's premature at this point. ③

She hears the discussion and chooses a modified radical mastectomy. You are now in the operating room. Visualize the operation. Tell me how you do the modified radical mastectomy.

I try to develop skin flaps at least 2–3 cm in all directions around the neoplasm. I don't make a big deal about really thin flaps. I try to get into the plane between the subcutaneous fat in the breast tissue. In a nonobese patient, this plane is fairly easy to define. I use the electrocautery unit and cauterize vessels as we go along. Usually, if we stay in that plane, the bleeding is minimal, especially in a nonobese patient. I make the superior flap first, then an inferior flap. I start at about the left edge of the manubrium and proceed with medial-to-lateral removal of the breast along with the overlying fascia of the pectoralis. (Sometimes you have to secure with clips the intercostal vessels that penetrate the musculature, but most of the time these vessels also can be managed by using cautery.)

Once the breast is detached, I follow the lateral board of the pectoralis major up to the axillary sheath, which I incise. I have my assistant retract the tendon of the pectoralis minor medially and superiorly. Then I remove the axillary contents inferiorly from the medial to lateral aspect, identifying and preserving the long thoracic and thoracodorsal nerves. I make no effort to preserve the intercostal brachial nerve. I secure the branch of the axillary vein with hemoclips and divide it.

When I finish, I insert a solitary drain through the incision beneath and lateral to the mastectomy wound, placing it in the depths of the axilla, and then close the skin flaps with alternating skin staples and ¼-inch skin clips. I am not obsessed with closing subcutaneous fat—I think that's nonsense.

I leave the drainage catheter in place no longer than a week. I usually take it out in a week, even though about 20 or 30% of patients are going to get seromas. [4] Most seromas can be managed with periodic aspiration, and only a small percentage develop an axillary infection. But it seems to me that no matter how you treat the axilla, a number of patients are going to get seromas. I think the biggest risk of leaving the drainage catheter in place longer than a week is infection. I have seen severe axillary infections in patients in whom the catheter was left in place longer than a week, because it's a conduit for bacteria.

Surgical Observations

[1] Notice the emphasis on **discrete** mass. The surgeon mentions it twice in the first part of his discussion.

[2] The medicolegal implications of surgical practice rear their ugly head in this comment. Although the surgeon realizes, in the back of his mind, that the cytology is almost surely worthless, if the fluid is bloody he needs to send it for primarily medicolegal purposes.

3 This is an elegant discussion by the surgeon of what he talks about with the patient who has breast cancer. It is a fair, unbiased comparison of breast-conserving therapy with modified radical mastectomy, including the inconvenience of radiation therapy, which he balances against the fact that the radiation therapy does not entail systemic problems. It is interesting that he does not want to discuss adjuvant chemotherapy because it frequently confuses the patient (as well as medical students and residents!) to talk about adjuvant chemotherapy when the primary therapy is being considered.

4 In deciding to remove the drain at 1 week, the surgeon has considered the 20–30% incidence of seroma if drains are removed early, but he wants to avoid axillary infection enough that the 20–30% is acceptable. These actual numbers and the balancing of risks would be very difficult to glean from the surgical literature for use in typical decision-analysis techniques.

Expert surgeons know so much because they recognize scripts.

Cognitive Psychologist's Commentary:
Vague Breast Mass

An experienced surgeon has a large amount of knowledge. It covers the great variety of diseases and their presentations and the appropriate surgical or nonsurgical responses to each. It is remarkable that the appropriate knowledge comes to consciousness at the right time, so that it can control attention and behavior. The surgeon's ability to access this information arises from the basic nature of human memory. Two special characteristics of an expert's memory combine to make this possible.

First, there is the human capability to recognize or "know again" an extremely large number of things. For example, Standing, Conezio, and Haber[1] showed 2,500 photographs to college students for 10 seconds each, and then tested their memory by showing pairs of photos, one that had been shown before and one that had not. Students could recognize which photo they had seen before in about 90% of the pairs. People also can remember things experienced in the distant past. You can recognize the face of someone you went to school with or the telephone voice of someone you have not heard from in years. And you can recognize familiar objects from sketchy outlines (see box, next page).

Surgeons depend heavily on the ability to recognize. Such recognition occurs in the act of perceiving what is going on. Expert surgeons, while hearing and understanding the brief case description, are able to "tap into" or activate their knowledge about all such situations. When they hear "woman with mass in breast," the phrase immediately calls up their general knowledge about breast disease. In other words, all the categories,

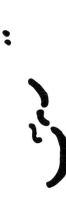

This sketchy outline is easily recognized as a violin. (From McCim RH,[2] with permission.)

distinctions, and procedures used to deal with such situations become active, ready to be used in further thinking about the new case. This activation is very rapid. For example, Elstein et al.[3] observed that doctors come up with a hypothesis during the first few sentences a patient says.

The second feature of expert knowledge and memory that is key for a surgeon's rapid access to appropriate knowledge is how the memory is organized. It may be described as a flexible script.[4,5] Like a script, it has a sequence of scenes that follow one after another. For example, in describing the operation the surgeon seems to divide it into four scenes: (1) the opening of the skin, (2) the removal of the breast, (3) the closing of the skin, and (4) the provision for aftercare. He knows these scenes very well. He can summarize them briefly, as here, or act within them for as long as required, as when actually performing the operation.

The surgeon's script is flexible. He knows many variations of each scene, all of which are covered by his script. For example, he talks about obese and nonobese patients. He knows he may see physical differences: for example, the planar surface, between the sub-cutaneous fat and the breast tissue, is more clearly visible in nonobese women. He knows to expect different reactions in obese and nonobese women and to be prepared to respond accordingly: thus, if he keeps the cut in this plane, there will be less bleeding, and because the plane is more difficult to see in obese women, they are likely to bleed more. Judging from the surgeon's spontaneous report, the knowledge of variations is organized within the general script of breast cancer rather than as separate scripts for obese and nonobese women.

After playing a scene one way, the surgeon can move smoothly to the next scene, adjusting so that it follows the first scene appropriately. This is visible in the statement, "Sometimes you have to secure with clips the intercostal vessels that penetrate the musculature, but most of the time these vessels can be managed by cautery." There are alternative ways to play each scene, depending on what the patient's body is like or on the surgeon's choice. Yet the script still marches on to its conclusion.

This scriptlike organization of the knowledge of how to do the operation enables surgeons to understand each other as they discuss past or future operations. Hearing the name of the condition, e.g., cancer of the breast, and a detail of a procedure in scene 3, a surgeon can use his or her knowledge of the "breast cancer script" to infer what probably happened in scene 2 or to ask about which procedural variant the operating surgeon chose to use in scene 4. For example, a surgeon might receive a phone call from a nurse: "Mrs. Jones had a mastectomy yesterday performed by your partner. She now has had 75 cc of blood out of her axillary drain in the past 2 hours." The surgeon may think, "My partner uses a hemoclip on a branch of the axillary vein. I wonder if it could have come off? Or is this just accumulated blood that has now appeared?" A mental script also serves as the basis for anticipation of what may happen in an operation one is about to perform and for planning the operation when there is an unusual variation in the initial situation.

The novice surgeon is faced with the task of acquiring knowledge that has both capabilities: (1) to recognize all the various illnesses/conditions and (2) to step through the sequence of scenes competently and flexibly. While the novice can try to attain the first capability through reading textbooks, the second capability can be acquired only through experience of cases.[5,6] It is as if there are two filing cabinets, one filled with medical facts and the other with knowledge that can be applied to the different types of patients. Although knowledge in the fact files is pertinent to the case files, students rarely make the needed connections unless someone shows them where to look in the fact file when they have a case file open. Thereafter, the connection is always available with that type of patient.[7]

1. Standing LG, Conezio J, Haber N: Perception and memory for pictures: Single-trial learning of 2500 visual stimuli. Psychonom Sci 19:73–74, 1970.
2. McCim RH: Thinking Visually: A Strategy Manual for Problem Solving. Belmont, CA, Lifetime Learning Publications, 1980, p 14.
3. Elstein AS, Schulman LS, Sprafka SA: Medical Problem-Solving: An Analysis of Clinical Reasoning. Cambridge, MA, Harvard University Press, 1978.
4. Schank RC, Riesbeck CK: Inside Computer Understanding: Five Programs Plus Miniatures. Hillsdale, NJ, Erlbaum, 1981.
5. Schmidt HG, Norman GR, Boshuizen HPA: A cognitive perspective on medical expertise: Theory and implications. Acad Med 65:611–621, 1990.
6. Patel VL, Groen GJ, Scott HM: Biomedical knowledge in explanations of clinical problems by medical students. Med Educ 22:398–406, 1988.
7. Abernathy CM, Hamm RM: Surgical Intuition. Philadelphia, PA, Hanley & Belfus, 1994, chapter 11.

8. LARGE BREAST MASS

A 41-year-old woman with a large mass in the upper quadrant of her breast has a negative mammogram, and ultrasound reveals that the mass is noncystic. You are examining her. What are you going to do?

If this is an asymmetric mass on physical examination and I'm convinced there is an abnormality, ☐ then it's important to know a number of things, such as family history. But you still come down to the basic question: to biopsy or not to biopsy. And if there's any question in my mind, I biopsy. ☒

Do you do a needle biopsy or an open biopsy?

If it's a diffuse nondescript mass, I do an open biopsy, because I don't want a sampling error.

Your biopsy comes back confirmatory for ductal carcinoma of the breast. You're talking to the patient about her diagnosis. What do you say to her?

We talk about treatment options, which depend largely on the size of the lesion. Basically, our first job is to control the primary lesion. Normally I like to screen these patients in advance, including chest x-ray, bone scans, liver functions, and so forth. Presuming these tests are all right, we have a lesion in the upper outer quadrant of the left breast that is infiltrating duct carcinoma.

There are two options: (1) a lumpectomy with axillary dissection and (2) a mastectomy. I would go into the pros and cons of both, and how they relate to the patient, her life, and her personal situation. This assumes that the tumor is small enough to allow me to do a lumpectomy with an axillary dissection. Personally I prefer to do the two procedures in continuity (particularly the upper outer quadrant lesions).

The patient chooses a modified radical mastectomy. Now you're in the operating room. Visualize the operation. Tell me how you do the modified radical mastectomy.

For an upper outer quadrant lesion I probably would do a modified Halsted incision. I like to create superior and inferior skin flaps, and I like to isolate the lesion with towels and so forth. I take the breast off the chest wall, and depending on how it situates itself—if it's really movable and nowhere near the pectoralis—I leave the fascia on top; if I'm concerned, then I'll take the fascia. Basically I take off the breast, leaving it hanging on the axilla, and then I do a modified axillary dissection. I leave both the pectoralis major and minor muscles and do an axillary cleanout in the standard fashion, preserving the long thoracic nerve and the thoracodorsal nerve. But I usually sacrifice the sensory nerve to the arm pit, the intercostal brachial nerve, and I close the wound over Hemovacs. In a 41-year-old patient one may give consideration to immediate reconstruction; again this is predicated on your previous talks with the patient and how she feels about it.

Surgical Observations

[1] The clinical suspicion begins the algorithm. The real question lies in the answer to "If I'm convinced there is abnormality"—which precedes entry into the algorithm.

[2] The system is loaded toward biopsy, but still *some* cases are not biopsied. Therefore, again, the question not answered by the algorithm (or textbook) is what triggers the clinician to biopsy or not to biopsy. Is it discreteness? Is it dominance? Is it slightly harder texture?

Expert surgeons' rules may not accurately describe how they think.

Cognitive Psychologist's Commentary: Large Breast Mass

The decision whether to biopsy a large breast mass, after negative mammogram and negative ultrasound, depends largely on the surgeon's judgment. This expert surgeon's explanation, "if there is any doubt, I biopsy," sheds little light on how that judgment is made. What exactly makes him doubt? And does he really biopsy if there is any doubt whatsoever—or does he balance the risks of undetected cancer with the sure costs of the procedure, which are greater with the more reliable open biopsy?

Psychological analysis often starts with a model describing processes that may occur in the mind. Figure 1 shows a simple model of how the surgeon may think about whether to biopsy. It takes the surgeon at his word: first he judges the amount of doubt; then he decides whether to biopsy, following the rule, "if there is any doubt (more than 0), then biopsy." This rule could easily be represented in a computer program.

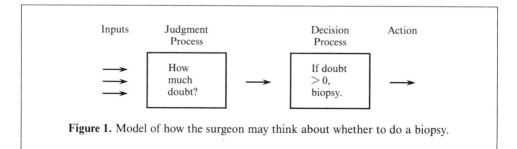

Figure 1. Model of how the surgeon may think about whether to do a biopsy.

But should we take the surgeon at his word? It is reasonable to assume he implicitly makes tradeoffs, because a biopsy, especially an open one, is not a trivial procedure. Let us imagine that we observed this surgeon and discovered that he biopsies 90% of all lumps in this situation (lumps of a certain size, with negative mammography and ultrasound). If a new, noninvasive, technique of proven equal accuracy were to become available, would he still use it on 90% of such patients? Or would he use it on 92%, 95%, 99%? If he would use the cost-free technique with a higher percentage of such lumps, then in a few cases of the 10% originally not biopsied, he had *some* doubt. It is not that the surgeon is dishonest when he describes his rule as "If in any doubt, biopsy." Rather, his judgment about whether there is any doubt is so tightly linked with the decision that it is hard to separate them. When the parameters of the decision change, his process of judgment also changes. We can change our model to reflect this (Fig. 2), adding an arrow from the decision box to the judgment box.

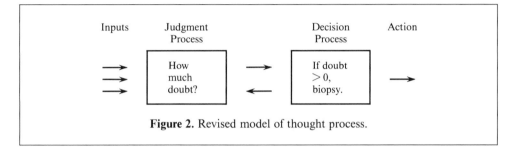

Figure 2. Revised model of thought process.

The additional arrow signifies that the surgeon's judgment process depends on the decision process. If the context of the decision were to change (e.g., if the cost of biopsy changed), then the judgment process also would change. If biopsies were less harmful, then the surgeon would be less reluctant to say doubt exists. This accounts for how the surgeon, still following the same rule ("If in any doubt, biopsy"), may shift from a biopsy rate of 90% to 95% for patients with this sort of lump if the cost of biopsies changed.[1]

At this point psychologists begin to disagree on how the model in the figure should be further specified to represent the interconnection we are talking about. Some may say that a threshold of doubt (T) must be exceeded before the surgeon acknowledges any doubt, even though he reports it as an absolute categorical judgment. Others may argue that the threshold applies to the *decision*, i.e., the decision rule is really "if doubt > T" for some T greater than 0 rather than "if doubt > 0." One way to avoid quibbling over details that are difficult to resolve is to collapse the process into one judgment–decision box. With such a "black box," we would talk only about how the output (the decision whether to biopsy) varies as a function of the inputs (e.g., information about the lump, the costs of biopsy).

The decision depends on experience. In a climate in which the doctor is blamed if a cancer is considered and missed, and biopsy is done if there is any doubt, it can be anticipated that the less experienced doctors will biopsy more often. The expert, then, uses his or her knowledge primarily to decide which of the lumps not to biopsy. A different master surgeon had this to say:

> Let's consider breasts. A lot of women out there have fibrous lumps in their breasts. Some doctors I know just say "I biopsy every one." But you need to exercise good judgment. I don't think it's fair to patients to biopsy every lump you see. You talk to those doctors and they say "I'm afraid of getting sued." When you start out in surgery you follow the algorithm, but as you gain more experience you deviate from it as appropriate.

What happens in the mind as one gains experience? The experts' judgments about which lumps not to biopsy are based on their own actual experience and on knowledge transmitted from others.

Experience. The experts themselves have felt the breast lumps and seen the subsequent findings on biopsy. They have made a correlation between the two, so that when the lump in a new patient feels like earlier lumps that were not cancerous, they can judge it as unlikely to be cancer. Managing these sensory impressions challenges one's ability to coordinate information. In fact, experimental studies (with simpler tasks, in controlled settings) have shown that people do not learn very well from outcome feedback: observing a series of events in which an initial appearance (such as the feel of a lump) is followed by an outcome (such as the result of a biopsy) does not allow them to learn what is associated with what.[2] They learn more quickly if you tell them the associations.

Knowledge from others. The other way to learn about the connection between the feel of breast masses and the probability of cancer (and hence about the usefulness of biopsy if other tests are negative) is through verbal communication with others. For this, of course, one must know the vocabulary for describing how the breast feels—e.g., the size, firmness, symmetry, or diffuseness of the mass (the same terms that one may use in learning from one's own experience). And someone has to have discovered previously the valid relations.

We know that valid relations can be discovered through scientific studies. But the community of practitioners offers another advantage: a larger number of observers multiplies the chance that an individual will discover valid relations. As the studies cited above showed, it is difficult for individuals to discover relations by trial and error. But there are probably a few surgeons who have had the right experience and the mind prepared to notice the relations. Once a relationship is noticed, others will recognize it in reflecting on their own experience, and then dissemination is a relatively easy matter. Of course, there is also the problem of false discovery and propagation of beliefs about relations that do not really exist.

Does it matter whether the judgments in the expert's mind are based on induction from his or her own experience or on communications from others? As long as the relations are valid, it should make no difference. Once the relations are learned and incorporated into the expert's automatic judgment processes, the judgment happens the same way whether it is based on personal experience or on shared knowledge. (See also the commentary on the Vague Breast Mass think-aloud, p. 31.)

---

1. Tierney WM, Miller ME, McDonald CJ: The effect on test ordering of informing physicians of the charges for outpatient diagnostic tests. N Engl J Med 322:1499–1504, 1990.
2. Hammond KR. Annotated bibliography on cognitive feedback (Report No. 269). Boulder, CO, Center for Research on Judgment and Policy, University of Colorado, 1987.
3. Hammond KR, Summers DA, Deane DH: Negative effects of outcome-feedback in multiple-cue probability learning. Organizational Behavior and Human Performance 9:30–34, 1973.

9. STAB WOUND TO CHEST

A 28-year-old man with a stab wound to the left chest in the midaxillary line, 6th intercostal space. His vital signs are pulse 120, blood pressure 120/80. What are your thoughts? What would you do?

The problem is that such patients may go into deep shock suddenly. First I would assume the worst, ① and secondly, I would put him somewhere where I can deal with the worst if it happens. The order of concerns is (1) the wound has hit the heart or part thereof and (2) it possibly hit the lung and then may go through the diaphragm and hit something subdiaphragmatic. I don't know the direction of the stab wound. I make a clinical decision as best I can along those lines.

If the patient remains stable, I have time to do a chest film and to insert a chest tube if that's appropriate. If he remains stable, I have time to go to the abdomen, do a peritoneal lavage, and look for evidence of penetration. If at any stage ② he becomes unstable, I react to the manner in which he became unstable, with the understanding that I would be quite happy to open up his chest very early on.

A left chest tube produces 400 cc of blood. Diagnostic peritoneal lavage (DPL) shows 3,000 red cells per cc. What are your thoughts? What would you do?

I would assume that the DPL is done according to our own recommendations, which include an open procedure and meticulous hemostasis. Therefore, we regard any red cells as evidence of peritoneal penetration in this situation and regard 3,000 cells as a requirement for laparotomy. Therefore, if I had cleared both the chest and the heart from evidence of further problems at the moment, I would proceed to a diagnostic laparotomy with the intention of clearing the diaphragm and peritoneal cavity.

While you are preparing the patient for laparotomy, another 1,000 cc of blood comes out the chest tube. You take him to the operating room, and first you explore the chest, finding an actively bleeding deep laceration of the left lower lung. Describe what you would do.

In the first instance, I would use a tamponade. I would make sure that the anesthesiologist had enough lines, enough time, and enough resuscitation to catch up and bring the patient back to hemodynamic stability. ③ At that stage, I would attempt to oversew the laceration. Does oversewing work?

Oversewing doesn't work. It is still bleeding.

I then attempt a partial lobectomy on that side.

Surgical Observations

[1] The surgeon's first thoughts are that the clinical picture in a patient with a stab wound to the chest often does not give clues as soon as in most patients with hemorrhagic shock injuries. Paramount in his thoughts is "assume the worst."

[2] Note the comment, "if he remains stable," which is repeated several times. The surgeon can make the decision to go to the operating room at any point during the actual algorithm he is using.

[3] This comment is almost identical to that made by another trauma surgeon in the Liver Laceration think-aloud, p. 142.

Thinking aloud prepares expert surgeons for the unexpected.

Cognitive Psychologist's Commentary: Stab Wound to Chest

The master trauma surgeon knows what is important here. He frames the situation with reference to the possibility that the patient may suddenly go into deep shock. He lists possible types of injury, in order of importance: "The order of concerns is (1) the wound hit the heart or part thereof and (2) it possibly hit the lung and then may go through the diaphragm and take something diaphragmatic."

This ordering is fundamental to how he thinks about the patient. For example, when told that both the chest tube and DPL produce blood, although he turned the discussion to the question of abdominal injury, still he maintained the priorities stated earlier: "if I had cleared both the chest and the heart from evidence of further problems at the moment, I would proceed to a diagnostic laparotomy with the intention of clearing the diaphragm and peritoneal cavity."

How important are the surgeon's expressions of the relative threat of the different possible injuries for his response to a particular patient? Some expert surgeons may rarely verbalize such considerations. Some experts, like this one, may say them aloud or to themselves every time.

We know that explicit verbal expression of such priorities is useful when surgeons are teaching students and residents and when surgeons are learning and need to work through the situation analytically.[1] But some experts may always verbalize the relative importance of different aspects of a situation, even long after they have attained expertise in the area.

Let us consider this surgeon's statements concerning the threats of chest versus abdominal injury and compare them with a photographer's statements about the lens opening, exposure duration, and film speed in planning and taking a picture. The expert photographer does not need to discuss these variables in most cases. He or she can just do it the usual way, reading the meter or letting the camera set the exposure automatically. Verbal statement of the lighting situation and the factors that the photographer controls facilitates the discovery of additional possibilities, the recognition of different effects that would not be discovered if the photographer merely followed the usual script. The habit of analysis of the exposure enables the photographer to get better shots by recognizing possibilities that are not immediately obvious. Similarly, the surgeon's explicit statement of the possible injuries and their relative threats provides a framework for decisions about diagnostic procedures and a readiness to respond to anything that may happen. It is a tool the surgeon uses to keep his mind ready to respond when the situation shifts from one script to another or beyond scripts.

Most of the time the photographer can use conventional exposures, and so discussion of the light is unnecessary. But if the subject offers a special opportunity, the photographer who has been talking about exposure will be ready to take advantage of it, whereas the photographer who has been following the script mindlessly will not.[2] Similarly, most of the time the surgeon's verbal expression of the relative importance of the various mechanisms of stab wounds will be redundant with the scripts for responding to stab wounds. But occasionally the situation will demand a quick shift between scripts or a response that the surgeon has never made before. If the surgeon has been stating the possibilities explicitly—naming and ordering the possible injuries to heart, lung, diaphragm, abdomen—the ideas, images, and responses will be actively in mind, so that an appropriate response can be made very rapidly if needed. If the surgeon has not been doing so, he or she will have to start thinking about the appropriate response from scratch and may not respond appropriately or quickly enough.

1. Abernathy CM, Hamm RM: Surgical Intuition. Philadelphia, PA, Hanley & Belfus, 1994, chapters 5 and 11.
2. Langer EJ: Mindfulness. Reading, MA, Addison-Wesley Publishing Company, 1989.

10. THORACIC OUTLET SYNDROME

If a patient has a history and physical exam consistent with a thoracic outlet syndrome, how would you manage it?

I'd have to be convinced. I'm not easily convinced that there is such a thing as thoracic outlet syndrome. ① Of the thousands and thousands of supposed cases that come through Denver, I've been convinced by only a few when I can demonstrate venous obstruction on a venogram. There are really two options. Personally, I'd do everything possible not to operate. It's always important to see if there is litigation. My experience has been that secondary gain is always involved with some syndromes. However, given that we've accepted the existence of thoracic outlet syndrome and have exercised the patient with no results, then it comes to a choice of scalenectomy or first rib resection. Personally I'm an advocate of first rib resection. But again, it's not a good case to present to me because I am from Missouri, so you have to "show me." ② I'm not so sure about this syndrome.

Surgical Observations

① Rather than talk about the textbook signs, symptoms, and therapy of thoracic outlet syndrome, the surgeon focuses on his nonbelief, his suspicion of the whole situation. He talks about such factors as secondary gain (even though he is not actually seeing a patient) and litigation.

② Textbooks seeking to define and distinguish all possible syndromes would not give such an overview, which needs to dominate the process. This demonstrates why these written scripts, if read by a learning or less experienced surgeon, are helpful in understanding what really is in a surgeon's mind as he or she thinks about a given clinical problem.

Can prejudice be based on probabilities?

Cognitive Psychologist's Commentary: Thoracic Outlet Syndrome

The expert's knowledge is organized as needed for use. In this surgeon's experience, almost every time the diagnosis of thoracic outlet syndrome is used, there is the possibility that the patient is malingering, or more charitably, that the patient's genuine suffering needs to be given a "hard" diagnostic label in order to qualify for reimbursement for care or time off work with pay. And even in a hypothetical case, with absolutely no evidence that such a process is going on, this suspicion is first in the surgeon's mind.

There is controversy about whether such a response is appropriate. What if someone really had the syndrome and came to the surgeon for help? Wouldn't he be an unfair or biased judge? Shouldn't the doctor judge each case on its merits alone?[1]

The surgeon refers to a hard sign that identifies the thoracic outlet syndrome for him: demonstration of venous obstruction on a venogram. Similarly, emergency physicians should be able to discern quickly that patients who walk into the emergency department with Munchhausen's syndrome need to be sent on their way. But sometimes there are false negatives, and in the climate described, this surgeon would not give the patient with thoracic outlet syndrome that was not clearly evident on venogram the benefit of the doubt.

Some doctors believe it their duty to treat each patient as unique and further believe that they can do so, attending only to the particular patient, not to the base rates. Although one can imagine programming a computer to "think" in this way, and although the intern combing the textbooks to find out what is wrong with a patient may think in this way, it is not plausible that an expert surgeon would be able to do so. The process of mental pattern recognition is based on experience. If the expert has seen many cases purporting to be thoracic outlet syndrome but has seldom found one that he or she considers "real," the expert will expect each new purported case to be something else.[2,3]

It would make little difference if the surgeon missed a true case of thoracic outlet syndrome because he or she expected it not to be real. Although the operation would not be done at this time, bringing relief, the chance of permanent injury is minimal. The time and vigor of the patient in pursuing treatment (with multiple visits and tests) are used to sort out the genuine cases. A related issue is the effect of annoyance and disbelief on an expert's thinking. Studies have shown powerful effects of expectations on various sorts of reasoning.[4] Certainly the expert who does not keep an open mind even in the face of strong expectations and makes no attempt to distinguish the real from the fake is not truly exercising his or her expertise.

---

1. Bar-Hillel M: The base-rate fallacy in probability judgments. Acta Psychol 44:211–233, 1980.
2. Rosenhan D: On being sane in insane places. Science 179:250–258, 1973.
3. Duffy TP: The red baron. N Engl J Med 327:408–411, 1992.
4. Rosenthal R, Jacobson L: Pygmalion in the Classroom. New York, Holt, Rinehart, & Winston, 1968.

11. LIVER METASTASES

A 48-year-old man underwent resection of a Dukes B2 left colon lesion 3 years ago. Preoperatively he had a CEA of 19, and then it went down to 1. During follow-up the CEA rose to 17. The gastroenterologist did a work-up. The CT scan shows a 5.0-cm solitary lesion in what appears to be the dome of the right lobe of the liver. The patient has no evidence of metastatic disease in his lungs on chest x-ray or CT scan. How would you handle the patient?

I assume that they also have scoped him to make sure that he has no intraluminal disease? And the time frame is 3 years? He's probably on the border in terms of patients who have early recurrences of hepatic metastases that clearly they did not have at the original surgery. These patients are most likely to have diffuse metastases on exploration. Two-and-a-half to 3 years—we presume that this is probably an isolated hepatic metastasis that over time has become obvious in terms of increasing CEA and visibility on scanning.

First, you want to make sure he has no other intraperitoneal disease. A laparoscopist can make sure that the patient has no other peritoneal seedings. If he clearly has an isolated hepatic metastasis and is 48 years old, we know his survival is going to be better with hepatic resection if he clearly has no other demonstrable disease. ⬜ Now the question comes down to how good we are at CT scanning or finding other hepatic metastases. MRI is not that much more sensitive in picking up metastases. Some think that the combination of both CT and MRI more clearly defines isolated lobar disease.

I would probably use intraoperative ultrasound, making sure that the patient has no other hepatic metastases.

At exploration, there is no other evidence of intraperitoneal disease. Intraoperative ultrasound suggests that all he has is a fairly large 5-cm tumor in the dome of his right lobe. Visualize and tell us technically how you would take out the tumor.

There are two types of hepatic resections you can do. The standard resection includes dissection of porta hepatis, with isolation and division of bile ducts, portal venous flow, and arterial input. But my experience has been that inflow occlusion in a patient who otherwise has normal liver function (that is, putting a clamp over the porta hepatis) certainly reduces the amount of blood loss so that you can then isolate the right hepatic artery, right duct, and so forth. Then you either finger-fracture, or use the ultrasonic dissector, isolating all the hepatic triads and the small vessels as you come across them. Basically, you are to do a right lobectomy because I assume that when you say in the dome, it probably is in the right lobe. The metastasis isn't close to the line, in the gallbladder bed, which divides the right lobe from the medial segment of the left lobe. You can dissect along that plane and reduce the blood loss significantly.

It used to be thought that the warm ischemia time for liver was probably on the order of 45 minutes, but a recent study of patients with similar hepatic metastases—in other words, no normal liver disease—showed that the warm ischemia time is much extended and may be as long a 1½–2 hours. This may not hold for patients who perhaps have chronic active hepatitis and cirrhosis.

You wouldn't cool him?

No, you don't need to cool him.

Surgical Observation

[1] The attending surgeon continually returns to the phrase, "if the patient has no other evidence of disease." In other words, he constantly challenges (with tests, examinations, and so forth) to see if indeed other metastases are present.

When experts look forward, they do not have to think hard about what to do.

Cognitive Psychologist's Commentary:
Liver Metastases

This think-aloud illustrates two features of expert thinking that cognitive psychologists have identified: experts spend a great deal of time figuring out the situation, and they work forward rather than backward.

Those with relatively little experience do a lot of exploring when they are working on a problem. They may start right in and then come up against a decision; thus they have to think hard about their various options. In contrast, experienced clinicians spend less time thinking about what to do and more time figuring out what is going on.[1] This is true in other domains as well. Physics professors spend relatively more time observing the given information than their students.[1,2] "Students who are successful at solving formal analogy problems frequently take more time to encode the initial problem information than do less successful problem solvers."[3] And the surgeon here devotes a lot of attention to making sure that there is no intraluminal or intraperitonial disease. The index of suspicion is high, for the doctor knows that this type of patient usually has widespread metastases.

Novices often approach problems by working backward from the goal. In contrast, experts start at the beginning, with steps that are related to the goal but that are done routinely because they are so well known. The goal is reached without the expert's needing to think hard about it. Whitehead overstates the point only slightly:

It is a profoundly erroneous truism, repeated by all copy-books and by eminent people when they are making speeches, that we should cultivate the habit of thinking of what we are doing. The precise opposite is the case. Civilization advances by extending the number of important operations which we can perform without thinking about them. Operations of thought are like cavalry charges in a battle—they must be strictly limited in number, they require fresh horses, and must only be made at decisive moments.[4]

This point is evident in the way the surgeon deals with bleeding in the liver. She does two things ahead of time that control it: clamps the porta hepatis and cuts in a place that minimizes blood loss. This is possible because the expert's knowledge is in the form of a script that allows her to predict what is likely to happen: the cancer would probably be away from the line that divides the right lobe of the liver from the medial segment of the left lobe; that line, therefore, would be a good place to dissect, reducing blood loss. The expert does not have to wait for the bleeding to start and then react to it; the script provides for steps to minimize bleeding before it starts.

---

1. Lesgold A: Problem solving. In Sternberg RJ, Smith EE (eds): The Psychology of Human Thought. New York, Cambridge University Press, 1988, pp 188–213.
2. Larkin JH, McDermott J, Simon DP, Simon HA: Expert and novice performance in solving physics problems. Science 208:1335–1342, 1980.
3. Bransford J, Sherwood R, Vye N, Rieser J: Teaching thinking and problem solving: Research foundations. Am Psychol 41:1078–1089, 1986.
4. Alfred North Whitehead, as quoted by John D. Barrow in Pi in the Sky: Counting, Thinking, and Being. Oxford, Oxford University Press. Quoted in turn as a "Vignette" in Science 260:833, 1992.

12. CANCER OF PANCREAS

A 71-year-old man with jaundice and a 10-lb weight loss has an elevated alkaline phosphatase and a bilirubin of 8. How would you proceed with this patient?

First, you've got to see if the patient has any history of GI symptoms or any symptoms compatible with biliary colic or the like. ☐ The scenario you have given probably points to a previously asymptomatic man with painless jaundice. The alkaline phosphatase is elevated, the bilirubin is 8. I presume the hepatocellular enzymes are only moderately elevated, ☒ and this leads to a virtually definite conclusion that he has obstructive jaundice. The first test that needs to be done is an abdominal ultrasound: it's cheap, it feels good, and nobody ever died from it.

The abdominal ultrasound shows gallstones and a dilated common duct.

I need another piece of information from the ultrasound: what is the condition of the pancreas, if it was visualized?

Nonvisualized.

So the patient has one of two conditions: either he has choledocholithiasis, which causes his obstructive jaundice, or he is one of the small percentage of patients with a neoplasm in the peripancreatic area and incidental gallstones. At this point I do not feel the need for any further diagnostic tests, provided I have a reliable history of no alcohol abuse. At this point I would go to the OR.

In the OR you find a somewhat diffuse mass about 4 cm in the head of the pancreas. You explore the abdomen and find no other abnormalities. What do you do then?

At this point, the assumption has to be that the patient has a neoplasm either in the pancreas or in one of the periampullary structures: duodenum, distal bile duct, or ampulla. If he is in good shape, you begin mobilization of the head of the pancreas.

How do you do that?

First, open the gastrocolic ligament widely. You perform a wide Kocher maneuver to expose the area at the head of the pancreas, which you manually assess for mobility on the mesentery vessels. You also look for any lymph nodes in this area. If there are such lymph nodes, you biopsy and send them for frozen section.

You don't see any large lymph nodes. You have mobilized the head of the pancreas, and you find this somewhat diffused 4-cm mass in the head of the pancreas.

And the man is 71 years old? At this point, I would proceed with a Whipple resection. If you insist on a tissue diagnosis first, you are going to face the problem of a false-negative diagnosis. ③

49

Visualize in your mind and tell us how you do the Whipple resection.

The man has gallstones, correct? ④ At this point, once I have mobilized the pancreas, I want to do a cholecystectomy and operative cholangiogram, looking at the common duct. If there are common duct stones along with the mass in the pancreas, I would do a cholecystectomy and exploration of the common bile duct (CBD). If CBD stones are present, I also would do transduodenal biopsies of the pancreas, because I am still concerned that this could be a neoplasm. If there are no stones in the common duct and he merely has gallstones and a mass in the pancreas, I would continue with the Whipple operation.

Visualize and tell us how you do that operation.

Once the gastrocolic ligament is open and the duodenum is mobilized, the first step is to encircle and dissect out the common bile duct. I'd use a vessel loop to do this and then dissect distally along the bile duct. This approach brings you to the gastroduodenal vessels, which will be ligated at this time. I would then go under the neck of the pancreas; I personally use a curved Satinsky clamp and very gently put a Penrose drain around the pancreas. At this point, I put dorsal and ventral sutures on either side of the neck of the pancreas and transect the pancreas with a pair of scissors. This creates a little problem with bleeding, and you have to oversew the pancreas with interrupted mattress sutures, being careful that you don't ligate the duct. To avoid that, I always put a cholangio catheter in the duct when I am putting in the mattress sutures so I can be sure that I haven't included the duct.

At this point, I disconnect the bile duct. I always do pylorus-sparing Whipple resections, so I fully mobilize and transect the pylorus with the gastrointestinal anastomosis (GIA) stapler and go to the ligament of Treitz. I transect the pylorus 6–8 inches beyond the ligament of Treitz with a GIA stapler and then take the entire jejunal mesentery vessel as far to the right as I can at that point, ligating both sides as I go. Then I pass a loop under the mesenteric vessels. This leaves the entire pancreas in your hand, along with the distal bile duct and the jejunum. The only thing you have to be careful of now is blunt dissection of the mesentery portal vein from the pancreas. There are 3 or 4 little vessels here, which I stick-tie. Then you have to be careful that you don't retract too hard to the right and really splay the supramesenteric artery over to the right. This artery can be included in the Whipple resection if you're indiscreet. I just take it between hemostats at this point. Usually within 10 minutes of reaching this point in the operation, you have the pancreas off.

And putting it together?

I oversew the end of the jejunum, which is closed already. I mobilize the distal pancreas about 3 cm on its undersurface so that I have plenty of pancreas to work with (I am doing pancreatic gastrostomies now). I fix the pancreas to the under-surface, the back surface, and the antrum of the stomach. I make a small hole there, into which I invaginate the entire 3 cm of pancreas, and put some circumferential stitches so that the pancreas is dangled into the stomach. This is virtually 100% leak-proof. Then I do an end-to-side cholejejunostomy, and my last anastomosis is an end-to-side duodenojejunostomy immediately distal to the pylorus.

Surgical Observations

1. In this particular clinical setting the surgeon believes that the history is going to be very important in giving the direction of the work-up. This is not true in all surgical problems. He emphasizes that he is definitely going to take the time to find out the history of the jaundice, the weight loss, and other gastrointestinal problems.

2. The surgeon is willing to accept a "moderate" elevation of the hepatocellular enzymes without giving it any diagnostic value at all in the work-up of the patient. In other words, he has reset the norms in this clinical setting.

3. The surgeon has previously thought out what he is going to do if he does not have an "easy biopsy" or a false-negative biopsy.

4. The surgeon asked in his own mind whether the patient has gallstones. His questions reveal what is important. In this instance, he has to think about how useful the gallbladder may or may not be in doing this procedure. Once he realizes the patient has a gallbladder with gallstones, he proceeds with cholecystectomy and moves on. What follows is an excellent discussion of the technical aspects of a Whipple procedure.

Expert surgeons have "action" hypotheses.

Cognitive Psychologist's Commentary:
Cancer of Pancreas

Expert surgeons make decisions rapidly. The basis for the decisions is seldom fully articulated, but in this transcript the surgeon explains the strategy behind two decisions.

In the first of these decisions, after learning that the abdominal ultrasound shows gallstones and a dilated common duct, the surgeon decided to go to the operating room. He did not know whether the patient had choledocholithiasis or a neoplasm, but it did not matter. "At this point I do not feel the need for any further diagnostic tests provided I have a reliable history of no alcohol abuse. At this point I would go to the OR."

Experienced surgeons frequently do not bother to make a diagnostic decision if it would make no difference in the decision whether to operate. They can justify this practice by reference to each of the possible diseases, as a surgeon may vividly recall from his residency (see box). In sum, if an operation is appropriate if each possible diagnosis were true, then an operation is appropriate. It is not necessary to spend time, effort, or money trying to figure out a precise diagnosis before the operation. And, of course, the surgeon will acquire much information in the operating room; thus an operation represents a way to solve the diagnostic problem.

> What do you do if a mass in the cecum is a cancer?
>
> Operate.
>
> And what do you do if a mass in the cecum is an ameboma?
>
> Operate.
>
> And what do you do if a mass in the cecum is the appendix?
>
> Operate.
>
> So what do you do with a mass in the cecum?
>
> Operate!

While experienced surgeons are comfortable deciding to operate in the absence of an established diagnosis, nonsurgeons and inexperienced surgeons frequently hesitate and seek more information. There are many reasons for this. First is a desire for certainty.[1] Doctors in all specialties often feel a need to know what disease the patient really has, even when it would make no difference in treatment. Another issue is control over the patient. Whereas the surgeon keeps a patient that is going to the OR, for doctors in other specialties the decision to operate means that they lose the patient to the surgeon. The other doctor will no longer be involved in the primary decision making and will not be able to complete the intellectual problem that the patient posed.

A second reason for seeking a sure diagnosis before surgery is the novice surgeon's lack of knowledge and confidence. The expert surgeon has experienced many similar cases, gone through all the possibilities repeatedly, and confirmed his or her expectations in the operating room with patients that present with such symptoms. The novice surgeon knows the pertinent diseases but has doubts about the thoroughness of his or her information search: "Have I missed a possible disease? Is there some test that I don't know about that would clear this up and spare the patient an unnecessary operation?" Ordering additional diagnostic procedures is a way to gain both information that may be useful and a little time to mull over the situation.

And in some cases there is a rush to surgery when the patient might as well have waited. Here the surgeon has induced the pain and expense of surgery unnecessarily, a misapplication of the usually reasonable response of operating when an exact diagnosis is not necessary. Determining whether it is appropriate to operate without an established diagnosis is a difficult matter of judgment.[2] As their experience accumulates and as new techniques and new information become available, individual surgeons need to criticize and revise the patterns they recognize as justifying operations without diagnoses.

Objectivity in evaluating performance in each case requires attention not only to operative outcome (success/failure) but also to the surgeon's cognition. Was cognition clear at each stage? How was the surgeon misled? How would the surgeon avoid the mistakes in the next similar case? The surgical mortality and morbidity rounds offer the opportunity for such an objective review, as long as they provide an environment in which there is no economic or ego threat; that is, in which competing surgeons will not gain a monetary advantage by watching their colleagues expose their thinking processes.

The second interesting decision occurred in the OR, after a mass in the head of the pancreas was discovered and no large lymph nodes were found. The surgeon decided to proceed with a Whipple resection rather than to take a tissue sample from the mass for diagnosis: "If you insist on a tissue diagnosis first, you are going to face the problem of a false-negative diagnosis."

There is already sufficient grounds to take out the pancreas, based on the probability of cancer. If the tissue were tested and came back negative for cancer, the surgeon may feel compelled not to take it out or at least feel the need to justify the decision to take it out in the face of potentially unreliable evidence that the excision is unnecessary. To avoid this uncomfortable situation, he simply does not get the test in the middle of the operation.

In this situation the surgeon experiences information pertinent to a diagnosis as potentially harmful, something to be avoided. This can be compared with the first decision we discussed, in which the diagnostic information was considered irrelevant, something unnecessary to seek. Both views reflect the expert surgeon's deep knowledge of the cost and value of potential information and its relevance to the possible actions that the surgeon can take.

---

1. Bursztajn H, Feinbloom RI, Hamm RM, Brodsky A: Medical Choices, Medical Chances. New York, Routledge, 1990.
2. Abernathy CM, Hamm RM: Surgical Intuition. Philadelphia, PA, Hanley & Belfus, 1994, chapter 8.

13. MASS IN PANCREAS

You just opened the abdomen of a 62-year-old woman with gallstones on whom you are operating for presumed chronic cholecystitis. On exploring the abdomen you feel a 4–5-cm vague mass in the head of the pancreas.

I need to determine if it is rockhard or if it is just pancreatitis. There are stones in the gallbladder, so the mass could be a common duct stone. I would feel now for any enlarged nodes in the region, then reexplore the abdomen to see if there are tiny metastases in the liver on the peritoneal surface or anywhere else. □

You don't feel any metastases.

I would Kocherize the duodenum to get my fingers underneath the mass, with my thumb on top and my fingers underneath the duodenum and behind the pancreas.

It is definitely a mass, but it is poorly defined.

I see two choices for biopsy: insertion of a Travenol needle directly into the pancreas or right through both walls of the duodenum from a lateral approach. I try to avoid piercing the common duct. I would look at the common duct now and dissect the material over it. I would not take out the gallbladder until I knew the diameter of the common duct, because I may need the gallbladder to divert the biliary tract if the common duct is small.

The common duct looks to be about 1 cm in diameter, just on the borderline of being enlarged.

I would try to get a cholangiogram in some way. I don't think I would want to get it through the cystic duct, because I would need to keep everything intact in case I need the gallbladder. Because I am sure now that there is a mass in the pancreas, although I'm still not sure if it is pancreatitis or not, I would stick a Travenol needle—one stick at a time—into the head of the pancreas—into the hardest part of the mass—to see if I can get a diagnosis. I would freeze each stick one at a time. I want to see if the results are negative. Having done that, I would try to do a cholangiogram through the gallbladder, realizing that it is going to take a lot of dye to fill the gallbladder. I would have to try to position things so that the gallbladder dye doesn't obscure the distal duct. I would stick a needle in the gallbladder in an area I probably would use for an anastomosis (in the dome).

The cholangiogram shows what seems to be tumor at the distal duct. The frozen section shows an adenocarcinoma of the pancreas.

I know the cholangiogram is not 100% reliable. Now I would begin to ease my finger down along the posterior surface of the tumor, which I have now dissected out, to see if it is stuck to the portal vein. I also would isolate the superior mesenteric vein inferior to the pancreas and the superior mesenteric artery and begin to dissect out these areas. If they are free of tumor, I would now know that the tumor is probably resectable.

Surgical Observation

[1] The surgeon has been surprised by the mass in the pancreas in what he thought would be a routine cholecystectomy. He therefore switches gears and begins looking around for a lot of information he ordinarily wouldn't look for. He asks whether any nodes are enlarged and reexplores for tiny metastases that he may have overlooked initially. He talks about visualizing several things in his "mind's eye." He tries to visualize how to avoid piercing the common duct when he is inserting the Travenol needle. And he visualizes the "feel" of the mass between his thumb and fingers after he has Kocherized the duodenum. He is actually visualizing the operation, even though he is simply talking about it in this think-aloud.

The expert surgeon relies on "knowing-in-action."

Cognitive Psychologist's Commentary: Mass in Pancreas

In this think-aloud the surgeon attempts to present visual and tactile imagery as he focuses on the details of the manipulations. The resulting account is given almost entirely in concrete terms. It focuses on what the organs are imagined to feel like ("rockhard" pancreas), on actions that would be done in exploring (feeling for nodes) or operating (positioning things so that the gallbladder dye doesn't obscure the distal duct). Of interest, although the surgeon was "seeing" everything he talked about, no explicitly visual statements were made, such as a description of how an organ looked.

Although the surgeon is simply "talking about organs" and does not seem to invoke any higher reasoning, still much knowledge and thinking are involved here. Strategies, though stated in concrete terms, reflect sophisticated considerations and experience ("I would not take out the gallbladder until I knew the diameter of the common duct, because I may need the gallbladder to divert the biliary tract if the common duct is small."). As Ryle observed, "When I am doing something intelligently, I am doing one thing, not two."[1]

This thinking is what Schon describes as "knowing-in-action." We can recognize things, make judgments, and do actions spontaneously without thinking about what we are doing. "We are often unaware of having learned to do these things; we simply find ourselves doing them. . . . In some cases, we were once aware of the understandings which were subsequently internalized in our feelings for the stuff of action. In other cases, we may never have been aware of them. In both cases, however, we are usually unable to describe the knowing which our action reveals."[2]

When confronted with difficult situations, involving "complexity, uncertainty, instability, uniqueness, and value conflict,"[3] people who usually rely on "knowing-in-action" have to reflect on what they are doing, as they do it. In such situations, problems are not so much solved, as set: "the decision to be made, the ends to be achieved, and the means which may be chosen" are defined. "Problem setting is a process in which, interactively, we *name* the things to which we will attend and *frame* the context in which we will attend to them."[4] Thus, the expert surgeon's knowledge enables him to go immediately to the difficulties that would be presented by a mass in the pancreas, to define the problems that underlie these difficulties, and to sketch an approach to solving the problems, all the while speaking very concretely.

---

1. Ryle G: On knowing how and knowing that. In The Concept of Mind. London, Hutcheson, 1949, p 32.
2. Schon DA: From technical rationality to reflection-in-action. In Dowie J, Elstein A (eds): Professional Judgment: A Reader in Clinical Decision Making. Cambridge, Cambridge University Press, 1988, p 71.
3. Schon, p 69.
4. Schon, p 66.

14. POSTCHOLECYSTECTOMY DUCT INJURY

A 30-year-old woman had a laparoscopic cholecystectomy for acute cholecystitis 6 weeks previously. She is now jaundiced with a bilirubin of 14 and an alkaline phosphatase of 350. AST and ALT are normal. What are your thoughts? What work-up would you use?

You would have to be concerned that you either injured her common duct or left behind a stone in the bile duct. She needs endoscopic retrograde cholangiopancreatography (ERCP) as the next step, which would be diagnostic and potentially therapeutic.

They are unable to do an ERCP. What will you do now?

I would do a transhepatic cholangiogram in an attempt to define where the problem was. Then she will have to have an operation.

A percutaneous transhepatic cholangiogram shows several clips at the area of the cystic duct stump with a 0.5-cm narrowing of the common duct adjacent to the clips. What do you do?

I am trying to visualize what you just told me. You would have to assume a duct injury. I think I would operate on the patient.

Describe what you would do in the operation.

You have to figure out what is wrong. The patient is strictured. You probably have a common duct injury from the procedure itself. It may be as simple as the fact that you put the clips too close to the common bile duct, and you may be able to alleviate the problem by removing them and closing over the cystic duct. If the duct has been significantly injured (cut in two), it will have to be repaired, probably with a Roux-en-Y choledochojejunostomy as opposed to a direct repair by putting the two ends of the duct together. It's hard for me to visualize the problem, but you have to find out what's wrong, and you have to operate to do it. Then you have to make the appropriate repair. The patient needs an operation. [1]

Surgical Observation

[1] The surgeon is very comfortable in this scenario and has obviously faced this problem several times before and thought it out. He doesn't think endoscopy is of much value and does not mention any work-up that a less experienced surgeon or resident may be tempted to order at this time. The scenario deliberately did not give the surgeon an x-ray that showed the problem but made him visualize at several points what the problem was, what he may encounter in the OR, and so forth. He covers several possible types of injury to the duct and how he would fix them and finally reiterates the "bottom line"—the patient needs an operation, and some of what is done is going to be determined in the OR.

Visualization is a tool in surgical decision making.

Cognitive Psychologist's Commentary: Postcholecystectomy Duct Injury

Given a description of postoperative complications, the surgeon tries to visualize what went wrong. He would prefer ERCP, with its superior visualization and the possibility of inserting instruments, over the static image of the cholangiogram. If it were his own operation, he also might "rewind the video tape,"[1] recalling the operation to see if any details of the procedure could explain what is happening now.

Given a verbal description of the results of the cholangiogram, the surgeon needs time to visualize them, to create an image of the patient's organs after cholecystectomy. Knowledge from a variety of sources goes into this visualization: knowledge of the normal anatomy of the organs, the disease that led to the original operation and the typical efficacy of that operation, and the procedures used when the gallbladder is removed via laparoscope as opposed to an open operation. It takes time to construct a full visualization. This is not due just to the fact that the surgeon was not offered an x-ray, for it takes time to interpret an x-ray image too.[2]

The surgeon did not get a complete picture of exactly what had happened, but could assume it was a duct injury and therefore an operation is necessary. In surgery the decision to operate often precedes the diagnosis (see Cancer of Pancreas think-aloud). Not until the operation can the problem be seen; then the appropriate response to the problem will be immediately available. This holds for open procedures as well as for endoscopic ones—as the surgeon notes, the ERCP can be "diagnostic and potentially therapeutic."

Before x-rays, visualization depended on opening the patient. X-rays and other remote visualization techniques allowed a separation between the seeing and the doing, which allowed the surgeon to do more diagnosis prior to surgery. Currently, endoscopic techniques provide good visualization along with the capability to insert instruments, allowing the decision "to operate" again to precede the diagnosis.

---

1. Abernathy CM, Hamm RM: Surgical Intuition. Philadelphia, PA, Hanley & Belfus, 1994, chapter 10.
2. Lesgold A, Rubinson H, Feltovich P, et al: Expertise in a complex skill: Diagnosing x-ray pictures. In Chi MTH, Glaser R, Farr M (eds): The Nature of Expertise. Hillsdale, NJ, Erlbaum, 1988.

15. MELENA

A 55-year-old man presents with gross melena. Four units of blood are required to restore his blood pressure to normal. Endoscopy demonstrates a posterior duodenal ulcer with an oozing vessel in the base. What are your thoughts?

Endoscopy has already revealed the presence of a bleeding duodenal ulcer. The endoscopist will try to stop the bleeding either with a laser or a cautery at that time. He's already received how much blood?

Four units of blood.

At age 55, if he didn't stop bleeding with four units of blood, I would take him to surgery. I would do a vagotomy, oversew the bleeding ulcer, and do a pyloroplasty. ☐1

Twenty-four hours after surgery the nasogastric tube drainage becomes grossly bloody, and the patient requires 4 units of blood over 3 hours to maintain his blood pressure. What now?

I would have the patient rescoped and see if the bleeding is at the same source as originally, as most likely it would be. If it continues bleeding, I would return the patient to surgery, and at this time I would do an antrectomy, resecting the lower part of his stomach, and probably a Billroth I, if possible, or, if not, a Billroth II procedure. ☐2

Surgical Observations

☐1 This highly experienced surgeon has a trigger point for the operating room, depending on the amount of blood that has been needed to maintain the patient's vital signs. When asked specifically after this think-aloud how many units defined the trigger point, he was vague. The experienced surgeon often will not have a 3-unit, 4-unit, or 5-unit rule; rather, a more complex decision is made, taking into account what time period is involved, how active the bleeding appears (that is, is the nasogastric tube red), and the frailty of the patient. Thus, the surgeon did make a decision in the think-aloud protocol, but when pressed specifically on how he made that decision, he does not invoke the kind of rules that appear in the surgical literature.

☐2 In a patient who bleeds postoperatively the surgeon has a clear concise plan. He didn't fumble with his thoughts. He may consider other parameters, but basically everything he does is going to be laid within the framework that he outlines here.

Knowledge, not short-term memory, is the expert's strength.

Cognitive Psychologist's Commentary: Melena

In the expert's thinking about the initial presentation of the patient, an everyday frailty of human memory is revealed. He forgot an important detail from the initial paragraph and had to ask for it to be repeated. This reveals something about the sequence of the surgeon's thoughts—the amount of blood transfused was not the first thing he attended to. Rather, the first mental task was constructing the big picture, thinking about the "posterior duodenal ulcer with oozing vessel as revealed by endoscopy," and connecting this to his knowledge of the disease in his mental script. By the time the surgeon had considered an important implication—that the endoscopist had probably tried to stop the bleeding—the information about the amount of blood that the patient had required has slipped from short-term memory.

But now the surgeon needs this information. His initial representation of the patient's problem is the general pattern of duodenal ulcer, but he needs to adjust it for this particular patient. The amount of blood loss is key to this refining, and it is at this point that the surgeon asks for it to be repeated.

The surgeon's decision to operate is based on the amount of blood loss and several other factors, as noted in the surgical observations. Knowledge about how to make this decision is part of the surgeon's script, a complex body of knowledge that has become compiled into an efficient and automatic response.[1] It is frequently difficult for experts to explain their compiled knowledge, as it is for this surgeon.

Because the decision depends on several factors simultaneously, it is difficult to reduce it to a simple rule, e.g., if four units of blood are lost, the ulcer must be operated on. Such a rule does not consider the other factors. A complex set of rules could be written to cover the ways the decision depends not only on the amount of blood loss but on its history, its current activity, and the patient's frailty. However, the surgeon probably is not explicitly aware of such complex rules when he thinks about posterior duodenal ulcers. And if the surgeon does not routinely express his knowledge in such a form, as in teaching, his answer would probably be inaccurate or incomplete if you asked him to report his rules.

A computer "expert system" based on such a report would have the same faults. There are techniques that expert system builders can use to try to tease out the expert's never-verbalized knowledge in this sort of situation, but they require a certain amount of tolerance and cooperation from the expert.[2]

1. Abernathy CM, Hamm RM: Surgical Intuition. Philadelphia, PA, Hanley & Belfus, 1994, chapter 4.
2. Hamm R: Modeling expert forecasting knowledge for incorporation in expert systems. J Forecasting 12:117–137, 1993.

16. ADENOCARCINOMA OF STOMACH

A 62-year-old man has noted persistent epigastric pain for 3 months. He is otherwise asymptomatic. Physical examination and routine blood tests are normal. Endoscopy reveals an ulcerating lesion on the lesser curvature of the stomach proximal to the incisura. Biopsy shows adenocarcinoma. How would you manage this patient?

This patient, with a proven carcinoma of the stomach, is a surgical candidate. I would do a near-total gastrectomy, cleaning out the nodes as well as possible around the celiac vessels. Most likely I would do a Billroth II procedure.

Describe the way that you clean out the nodes and what judgments you make there.

Once you have the stomach divided proximally, you would drop down right into the gastrohepatic area, and depending on the operative findings, you would clean the vessels as well as possible from the left gastric and hepatic vessels as you resect that large segment of his stomach.

One week after surgery the patient still has a high nasogastric output, and Gastrografin swallow shows gastric outlet obstruction. What would be your plan?

At the time of surgery I probably would have placed a jejunal catheter for feeding purposes. I would keep his nutrition at an optimal level. Sometimes a high resection like this will not empty within the first week. I probably would have the patient endoscoped at the end of a week to see if there was any gross evidence of obstruction. But I probably would not return the patient for further operative procedure until I'd waited another 5–6 days. ☐

While you were waiting, what would you look for to decide whether you had to do the second operation?

His nutritional state, the volume of nasogastric suction, the way his heart, lungs, kidneys were doing postoperatively. The general condition would determine how long I may want to wait.

Surgical Observation

☐ Again, the surgeon has a fairly specific amount of time that he would wait postoperatively for the patient that appears to be still obstructed. He hedges in the next paragraph, depending on the general condition of the patient and other parameters.

Do "if-then" rules or statistical models more accurately describe an expert surgeon's intuitive judgment?

Cognitive Psychologist's Commentary: Adenocarcinoma of Stomach

The surgeon's decision whether to do a second operation in this sort of case is an example of an intuitive judgment based simultaneously on a number of patient features[1] (see Right Lower Right Quadrant Pain think-aloud, p. 85). Experts make these judgments rapidly and without words. If asked to explain the judgment, they can lay out the effect of different variables on their decisions, as this expert does in the last paragraph: the more of variable A, the more I lean to decision F; the worse his nutritional state, the more likely I am to operate.

Cognitive scientists have used two different formalisms to explain how experts make this type of judgment. One formalism is constructed from if-then rules. Thus, the relation may be expressed as follows: if there is gastric outlet obstruction 1 week after resection of adenocarcinoma, and the patient's nutritional state is poor, then reoperate. A large collection of such rules could "cover the waterfront," saying what the surgeon would do for every possible variation in the patient's condition after gastric resection.

The other formalism is a statistical model, in which a mathematical combination rule is derived with statistical methods from observations of many cases in which the surgeon's decision and all the relevant features of the patient are recorded. Specifically, the surgeon's decision is expressed as a function of the patient's characteristics.[1,2]

Which of these models is right—the collection of if-then rules or the mathematical combination of cues? Introspection cannot really decide this question for judgments that take place intuitively. An alternative approach is to use both kinds of models to describe the same judgments and see which approach is the more satisfactory.

There have been a limited number of comparisons of the accuracy of conditional rule (if-then) versus statistical representations of expert knowledge. Einhorn, Kleinmuntz, and Kleinmuntz[3] studied a clinical psychologist's judgments. They produced conditional rule models based on analysis of verbal protocols as well as statistical models based on judgments of cases. The statistical model of a clinical psychologist's judgments of the mental health of a set of college students described the psychologist's judgments better than the conditional rule model. Another comparison was provided by Larcker and Lessig.[4] The sets of rules derived from a guided, retrospective, process-tracing procedure predicted judgments somewhat better than a statistical model for 25 of 31 subjects. That rules were more accurate in one domain, averages in another, is perhaps a reflection of the different tasks.

Another question that psychologists have asked is whether these models perform as accurately as the experts on whom they are based. In the domain of weather forecasting, numerous comparisons have been made between the performance of expert weather forecasters, statistical models of the experts, and conditional rule based expert systems.[5,6] Generally, the statistical models of the experts and the rule-based expert systems performed at about the same level and were exceeded by only the best of the weather forecasters. The reader is invited to speculate about whether the findings in a study of surgical experts would be analogous.

1. Abernathy CM, Hamm RM: Surgical Intuition. Philadelphia, PA, Hanley & Belfus, 1994, chapter 8.
2. Speroff T, Connors AF Jr, Dawson NV: Lens model analysis of hemodynamic status in the critically ill. Med Decision Making 9:243–252, 1989.
3. Einhorn HJ, Kleinmuntz DN, Kleinmuntz B: Linear regression *and* process-tracing models in judgment. Psychol Rev 86:465–485, 1979.
4. Larcker DF, Lessig VP: An examination of the linear and retrospective process tracing approaches to judgment modeling. Accounting Rev 58:58–77, 1983.
5. Moninger WR, Flueck JA, Lusk C, Roberts WF: SHOOTOUT-89: A Comparative Evaluation of Knowledge-based Systems that Forecast Severe Weather. Uncertainty and AI Workshop, 1989, pp 265–271.
6. Stewart TR, Moninger WR, Grassia J, et al: Analysis of Expert Judgment and Skill in a Hail Forecasting Experiment. Boulder, CO, Center for Research on Judgment and Policy, University of Colorado, 1988.

17. GASTRIC ULCER

A 62-year-old man has noted persistent epigastric pain for 3 months. He is otherwise asymptomatic. Physical examination and routine blood tests are normal. Endoscopy reveals an ulcerating lesion on the lesser curvature of the stomach near the incisura. Biopsy is benign. How would you manage this case?

With a benign location for an ulcer, assuming it looks benign, the patient can be treated with hospitalization, at least to begin with, and histamine (H_2) blockers. But it's very important that he have follow-up in 6–8 weeks with a repeat endoscopy and a biopsy to make sure that the ulcer has resolved. ☐

Six weeks later the ulcer has not healed. Biopsy is benign. You decide you need to operate. How would you handle the operation?

I would probably do a subtotal gastrectomy, if I am certain the lesion is benign. If it's a real small ulcer, you can wedge it out, but depending on how much room you've got, the best operation would probably be a subtotal gastrectomy. ☑

What if the ulcer is high—1 inch below the gastroesophageal junction?

I would probably try to wedge it out up there so I didn't have to do a high proximal gastrectomy with an esophageal anastomosis, assuming that the process is benign. But if the ulcer is high enough, you're going to have to do a proximal gastrectomy.

One week after surgery the patient still has a high nasogastric output, and Gastrografin swallow shows gastric outlet obstruction. What would be your plan?

One week after surgery? Because they sometimes take 2 or 3 weeks to open up, I'd manage the patient conservatively. You could endoscope him and make sure that it was open—that is a possibility. But I would just leave the tube down and put him on total parenteral nutrition (TPN). This procedure will probably open the gastric outlet.

Surgical Observations

☐ Three different times in this scenario, the surgeon hedges on the possibility of a false-negative biopsy. He notes "benign location," "assuming it looks benign" (gross appearance), and a repeat biopsy in 6–8 weeks. Note that the algorithm for gastric ulcer, part of which is included here, includes biopsy only at the first step (Fig. 1).

Down the line on the benign side, the algorithm assumes that the biopsy is trustworthy. The written text accompanying the algorithm notes that endoscopic

Observations continued on next page.

visualization biopsy provides about an 85% accurate reflection of malignancy or benignancy. As in most algorithmic thinking, the 15% false-negative rate is not readdressed later, as the surgeon in this think-aloud script did several times.

2 The surgeon hedges on "how much room you've got," meaning how proximal the ulcer is. He has visualized in his mind a benign gastric ulcer operation and, without having any information on the exact location or size of the ulcer, he has hedged in his mind whether or not the ulcer will come out with a subtotal gastrectomy. In other words, he wants to make sure that he has the technical possibilities in mind as he considers an operation. These are the thoughts that he would have while seeing a patient in his office with a nonhealing ulcer.

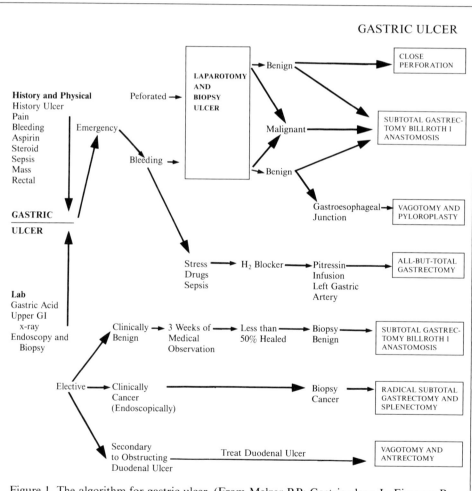

Figure 1. The algorithm for gastric ulcer. (From Melzer RB: Gastric ulcer. In Eiseman B, Wotkyns RS (eds): Surgical Decision Making. Philadelphia, W.B. Saunders, 1978, p 163, with permission.)

The expert surgeon is smarter than the algorithm.

Cognitive Psychologist's Commentary:
Gastric Ulcer

As the surgical commentator notes, the expert surgeon keeps in mind the possibility that a benign biopsy has missed cancer. This recognizes the fact that the endoscopic visualization biopsy returns a false-negative 15% of the time when the patient has stomach cancer. Although the surgeon may know the numbers for the false-negative rate, he may not think of the fact each time he bases an action on it (e.g., a repeat biopsy 6 weeks after the initial biopsy). The fact has had a role in the formation of the expert's script, but it does not need to be recalled explicitly when the script is used.[1,2,3] And, of course, the second biopsy is usually done not only because of the known false-negative rate, but because something has happened with the patient that makes it a little more likely that the first biopsy was false, such as persistent symptoms or a changing clinical picture.

Surgical algorithms are based on experts' practice—on the scripts of one or several surgeons. Therefore, one could revise the algorithm by Melzer[4] to include additional biopsies after the initial negative biopsy to cover the possibility that the first one was a false-negative. This revised algorithm, which now addresses the problem of the false-negative rate, would be atypical of most published algorithms but certainly within the realm of possibility.

Would such revisions, applied generally, make algorithms more satisfactory tools? Let us consider several aspects of this questions. First, would the surgeon whom we are taking as a model for the revised algorithm do it the same way with every patient? He may be more cautious with a brief description of a hypothetical patient than with a real patient, with whom he could use all his senses in making clinical observations. Moreover, his response to real patients would vary, for he may be less likely to seek a second biopsy at 6 weeks with one patient than with another—for example, if the pain resolves. If the addition of a repeat biopsy to an algorithm cannot be universal but must be contingent on other features of the patient, then the revision will make the algorithm more complex. Branches reflecting the surgeon's responses to the major patient variations also would increase the tree's arbitrariness if these responses reflect the surgeon's idiosyncrasies. The tree would be harder to use, less attractive, and more rigid. Perhaps, then, algorithms are best if incomplete yet simple, leaving some issues to the user's judgment.

One way to make trees deal with the possibility of false positives is to use decision analysis in their construction;[5] that is, to pose the general problem of the tradeoff between (1) the costs of the second biopsy after an initial negative biopsy and (2) the potential for saved lives and reduced suffering that the second biopsy offers. If the second biopsy proves cost-effective in general, it should be included in the algorithm. The result would be a more complex tree, still rigid, but now based on a general analysis rather than on one expert's clinical practice.

The expert surgeon may still need to override a decision-analytically constructed algorithm in response to his judgment of the patient's particular situation. However, such judgments also could be incorporated in an algorithm. A branch in the tree could depend on the results of an analysis with inputs including (1) the surgeon's judgments of the probability the patient has cancer, given his or her particular clinical course and the initial negative biopsy and possibly (2) estimates of the patient's tolerance for the risk of cancer and for uncertainty. This analysis could produce a numerical index that could be compared with a threshold value. Then the algorithm would branch on the basis of the index—if the index exceeds the threshold, the biopsy is repeated.[6,7]

In this way, the algorithm is made flexible to the surgeon's judgment of the situation at the cost of more complexity and the increased probability that surgeons would not use it because they don't want to make the required numerical judgments or compute the index. (Supplying a "default" choice would allow surgeons who don't want to compute the index to use the algorithm.) In addition, the algorithm would be vulnerable to becoming covertly outdated if later research shows the numerical assumptions underlying computation of the index to be incorrect.

Different yokes for different folks. Surgeons at different levels of experience would have different preferences for the amount of detail in the algorithms. Beginners may need simple trees so they can follow what others are doing and learn their scripts. Intermediate surgeons who know the general script may prefer guidance in the details. And the experts may just do without them, because they have well-learned scripts that cover the territory and provide flexible responses that an algorithm can provide only with great intellectual effort.

1. Anderson JR: Cognitive Psychology and Its Implications, 3rd ed. New York, W.H. Freeman, 1990.
2. Lesgold A: Problem solving. In Sternberg RJ, Smith EE (eds): The Psychology of Human Thought. New York, Cambridge University Press, 1988, pp 188–213.
3. See discussion of declarative versus compiled knowledge in Abernathy CM, Hamm RM: Surgical Intuition. Philadelphia, PA, Hanley & Belfus, 1994, chapter 4.
4. Melzer RB: Gastric ulcer. In Eiseman B, Wotkyns RS (eds): Surgical Decision Making. Philadelphia, W.B. Saunders, 1978, pp 162–163.
5. Abernathy CM, Hamm RM: Surgical Intuition. Philadelphia, PA, Hanley & Belfus, 1994, chapter 7.
6. Clarke JR, O'Donnell TF Jr: A scientific approach to surgical reasoning. VI. Thresholds and confidence. Theor Surg 6:177–183, 1991.
7. Weinstein MC, Fineberg HV, Elstein AS, et al: Clinical Decision Analysis. Philadelphia, W.B. Saunders, 1980.
8. Abernathy CM, Hamm RM: Surgical Intuition. Philadelphia, PA, Hanley & Belfus, 1994, chapter 11.

18. GASTRIC OUTLET OBSTRUCTION

The patient is a 42-year-old man with a 2-year history of increasing acid indigestion. He has had a recent increase of epigastric pain, and 8 days of progressively severe vomiting. Endoscopy reveals that the gastric outlet appears obstructed. No ulcer is seen. Upper GI studies show gastric outlet obstruction. What would you do?

In this patient the most likely diagnosis, although they haven't demonstrated it, is gastric outlet obstruction secondary to scarring from previous peptic ulcer disease. ☐ My surgical procedure would be an antrectomy with a vagotomy and a Billroth I procedure.

How long would you wait to operate on him?

If he is highly obstructed but in good shape otherwise, depending on his nutritional state, I wouldn't wait any longer than a few days. He should tolerate the procedure well and should have a relatively excellent outcome. ☐

At operation you see a huge dilated boggy stomach. What operation are you going to do? Visualize the procedure and tell step-by-step how you would do it.

I would proceed with what we were discussing. Possibly a large boggy stomach would require more than an antrectomy procedure. However, I think it still would be satisfactory to do the vagotomy and the antrectomy. With a large boggy stomach you're going to have stomach left. I'd still most likely continue with a Billroth I procedure.

On the eighth postoperative day the patient still has a high nasogastric output, and on upper GI study the contrast material remains in the stomach for several hours. What would you do? When would you reoperate?

Most likely I would give him a trial of metoclopramide to see if it would stimulate emptying of the stomach. I would maintain his nutrition with parenteral hyperalimentation because in a patient like this I would not expect a gastric stasis. Again I would have him endoscoped, and if nothing specific suggested any organic type of obstruction, I probably would wait another 5 or 6 days before contemplating further surgery.

What would you do at operation? Visualize and talk it through step by step.

If on the next operation there were no obvious organic reason for a delay in emptying the stomach, I would at that time convert him, probably from a Billroth I to a Billroth II procedure. ☐ If there had been any evidence or any suggestion of previous reflux in such a patient, on the second procedure I may consider constructing a Roux-en-Y gastrojejunostomy rather than a simple Billroth II procedure. But that decision would be determined by the individual patient.

Surgical Observations

1. The surgeon is always keeping an open mind, always ready to challenge what he currently believes to be true.

2. The experienced surgeon is able to prognosticate despite sketchy information.

3. The surgeon has a plan to convert to another type of drainage, almost no matter what is found, with the exception mentioned. Again he has a plan despite the limited patient information.

Experts' rules are based on recognition, then action.

Cognitive Psychologist's Commentary: Gastric Outlet Obstruction

The master surgeon, given a summary description of a patient, has to fill in possibilities. For example, he surmises that most likely the patient's gastric outlet obstruction is secondary to scarring from previous peptic ulcer disease. Given this assumption, he has in his knowledge an immediate response—antrectomy with a vagotomy and a Billroth I reconstruction.

Much of the surgeon's knowledge revealed here is in the form of rules based on categorical judgments: (1) if he is highly obstructed, if in good shape otherwise, depending on his nutritional state, wait no more than a few days, and (2) if on second operation there is no obvious organic reason for a delay in emptying the stomach, convert from Billroth I to Billroth II.

The expert speaks in rules. But does he really think in rules, or is it just a way to explain in words his thinking, which may take place without words?[1] Some cognitive scientists have taken seriously the idea that experts' knowledge takes the form of rules.[2,3] Experts have been asked to express their knowledge in the form of rules, and then computer programs have been built that can work with these rules and produce recommendations similar to those of the experts.[4,5] (See example, next page.)

Although if-then rules based on categorical perceptions can be used to represent expert knowledge sufficiently to support a computer program that simulates what they do, this does not prove that if-then rules are the only way that experts think. In particular, experts also show the ability to integrate information that can vary continuously, on several dimensions, into overall judgments.[7,8,9] And surely they can reason using the two forms of knowledge, categorical rules and continuous judgments, in combination (see also the think-aloud on Large Breast Mass, p. 35).

Example of a Rule in a Rule-based Expert System

This rule, from an expert system for managing ventilators (named VM), establishes a definition for stable hemodynamics:[6]

Rule: stable hemodynamics
Definition: defines stable hemodynamics based on blood pressures and heart rate
Applies to: patients on volume resuscitation, continuous mandatory ventilation (CMV), assist devices, T-piece
Comment: Look at mean arterial pressure for changes in blood pressure and systolic blood pressures for maximal pressures.

If

> heart rate is acceptable
> pulse rate does not change by 20 beats/minute in 15 minutes
> mean arterial pressure is acceptable
> mean arterial pressure does not change by 15 torr in 15 minutes
> systolic blood pressure is acceptable

Then

> the hemodynamics are stable.

1. Bereiter C: Implications of connectionism for thinking about rules. Educ Res 20(3):10–16, 1991.
2. Anderson JR: The Architecture of Cognition. Cambridge, MA, Harvard University Press, 1983.
3. Newell A: Unified Theories of Cognition. Cambridge, MA, Harvard University Press, 1990.
4. van Melle W: The structure of the MYCIN system. In Buchanan BG, Shortliffe EH (eds): Rule-Based Expert Systems: The MYCIN Experiments of the Stanford Heuristic Programming Project. Reading MA, Addison-Wesley, 1984, pp 67–77.
5. Clancey WJ: Details of the revised therapy algorithm. In Buchanan BG, Shortliffe EH (eds): Rule-Based Expert Systems: The MYCIN Experiments of the Stanford Heuristic Programming Project. Reading, MA: Addison-Wesley, 1984, pp 133–146.
6. Fagan LM, Kunz JC, Feigenbaum EA, Osborn JJ: Extensions to the rule-based formalism for a monitoring task. In Buchanan BG, Shortliffe EH (eds): Rule-Based Expert Systems: The MYCIN Experiments of the Stanford Heuristic Programming Project. Reading, MA, Addison-Wesley, 1984, pp 397–423.
7. Anderson NH: Information integration theory: A brief survey. In Krantz DH, Atkinson RC, Luce RD, Suppes P (eds): Measurement, Psychophysics, and Neural Information Processing, vol. 2. San Francisco, W.H. Freeman, 1974.
8. Hamm RM: Modeling expert forecasting knowledge for incorporation in expert systems. J Forecasting 12:117–137, 1993.
9. Abernathy CM, Hamm RM: Surgical Intuition. Philadelphia, PA, Hanley & Belfus, 1994, chapter 9.

19. SMALL BOWEL OBSTRUCTION WITH HYPOXIC EPISODE

You are called to see a 65-year-old man who has had one previous operation, and his abdominal film shows a partial small bowel obstruction. He has had crampy abdominal pain for 3 days. He had an appendectomy 15 years ago. Would you look at the film and tell me how you might start thinking about the patient?

Any time a patient who has had a prior operation comes into the hospital with crampy abdominal pain—there was not mention of nausea or constipation, but I suspect he may have either or both—your first diagnosis has to be bowel obstruction, presumably on the basis of adhesions. The other common cause, of course, is an external hernia. First you have to take a more complete history to find out if indeed this is just a 3-day illness. Or could it have been building up for a period of time, making one think that it might not be an acute small bowel obstruction? ☐

You take a more thorough history and determine it is an acute small bowel obstruction. On this basis you decide to take him to the OR, where you open up the abdomen and find massive dense adhesions. Tell me what you do in the OR.

We're presuming I went to the OR. In some patients with small bowel obstruction you may want to take a period of time for volume resuscitation. First, treat with nasogastric tube and see the response, because a certain percentage of patients with an adhesive small bowel obstruction will get better. Assuming that there were indications for surgery and we're now in the operating room, the first step is choice of incision, which in small bowel obstruction is a critical decision. If the patient's only prior incision is an appendectomy, you have the options of either a vertical midline incision or—as I would prefer—a transverse incision either immediately above or below the umbilicus, depending upon his body habitus. Through a transverse incision, I would open the peritoneal cavity. Now I am faced with dense adhesions. You proceed to dissect the peritoneal cavity.

How do you do that?

It's a two-person job. My preference is to expose for the person with the scissors. I find that it is much easier for a resident to dissect what I am displaying than vice versa, because I have some plan as to where I am going and where I need to be. I think the operation proceeds more expeditiously when I serve as the first assistant.

You're dissecting along and suddenly notice that you have taken off a fair amount of serosa from the small bowel.

That can happen, but the mere fact that it happens doesn't mean it needs to be repaired. The issue is not whether the bowel is de-serosed, in which case it should be left as is and not "re-serosed" because this leads to further adhesion formation. The issue really is whether mucosa is visible. If so, those areas have to be repaired as they are encountered, and I would repair them at the time rather than wait until the end of the operation. ② Sometimes there is a tendency to miss some of the small areas at the conclusion of the operation. Basically, we're heading toward the right lower quadrant because that's where his adhesive small bowel obstruction is going to be. ③ So most of the adhesions will be on that side, probably stuck to the peritoneum on the anterior abdominal wall, maybe to the area of the pelvis and the cecum.

You finish dissecting out the small bowel and find an area of moderately dilated bowel tapering into an area of decompressed bowel but no really dramatic size difference. What then?

This is a problem. In the most simple circumstance you find a definite are of obstruction with dilated proximal bowel and decompressed distal bowel. Then you merely lyse the adhesion and leave the remainder of the adhesions intact in the peritoneal cavity. In the picture you're drawing, you don't sound convinced that you've actually visualized the point of obstruction. Given that circumstance, you have to dissect the entire peritoneal cavity from the ligament of Treitz to the ileocecal valve until you have assured yourself that there are no hidden areas of small bowel obstruction.

You did that. On the second postoperative day, the resident tells you that the patient has had some right-sided pleuritic chest pain, including a hypoxic episode with ABGs down to 50 for about 30 minutes. He's off the ventilator, his chest x-ray shows bilateral fluffy infiltrates, and his EKG is normal.

In the first place, you don't rush to the assumption that this represents a pulmonary embolus. ④ The differential diagnosis in this patient would range from pneumonia to myocardial infarction to pulmonary embolus—and possibly even a subdiaphragmatic collection abscess causing referred pain. So the first thing I would do is to put oxygen on the patient. Before I did anything else, I'd give him a bolus of 10,000 units of heparin. ⑤ This isn't goint to harm any patient who doesn't have a pulmonary embolus. If indeed he does have a pulmonary embolus, you would institute treatment at the earliest possible time.

The EKG is normal and the blood gases showed a PO_2 of 50, which is compatible with a pulmonary embolus.

In this case you need to know definitively. I would skip the ventilation-perfusion scan in this patient, ⑥ because we know that he has an abnormal chest x-ray. Chances are that the ventilation-perfusion scan is going to be abnormal on the right side, and that's going to leave you dangling. I would proceed directly to pulmonary angiography after I instituted oxygen and heparin therapy.

Surgical Observations

① The surgeon creates a simple differential diagnosis, basically between a flu-like syndrome or 3-day gastroenteritis versus a small bowel obstruction. The many other illnesses and problems that could present in similar ways basically included within those two categories or ignored.

Observations continued on next page.

2 An important surgical point! Basically, the surgeon is saying, "you will forget most things at the end of a case that you told yourself during the case to remember." The surgeon emphasizes doing the things that need to be done *at the time* rather than waiting for the end of the operation. This also applies to removing lap pads and so forth.

3 The surgeon realizes that the right lower quadrant is by far the most likely location of the problem. he is going to focus on that area throughout the dissection procedure.

4 With the postoperative complication, the surgeon's first thought is not to jump to the diagnosis of a pulmonary embolus.

5 Subsequently, after talking about a brief but accurate differential diagnosis, he treats the patient as if it is a pulmonary embolus, realizing the chances are low but mentioning that the bolus of heparin has low morbidity.

6 This statement shows the very low dlinically applicable knowledge that the surgeon believes he can obtain from the ventilation-perfusion scan. He uses "surgical reasoning" to go directly to the test that will be critical for making the next decision.

Experts consider disease frequency when recognizing diseases.

Cognitive Psychologist's Commentary: Small Bowel Obstruction with Hypoxic Episode

The surgeon's thoughts reveal a series of intellectual tasks, done so rapidly that only their result is evident. These include the naming of the likely hypotheses, the identification of evidence that would differentiate between the hypotheses, the formation of new plans when an accident (denudation of serosa) or obstacle (failure to find obvious blockage of small bowel) is encountered, and the response to the respiratory difficulties on the following day. What kinds of cognitive process may allow these tasks to be done so accurately and rapidly?

The surgeon rapidly identified two hypotheses, small bowel obstruction secondary to adhesions or secondary to external hernia. If a conventional computer program were to seek the hypotheses that best account fdor the patient's symptoms, it would have to search through a large database of possible patterns to find ones that matched or partially matched the given information. A computer could produce a response as quick as the surgeon's only by (1) making the comparisons very rapidly, (2) doing more than one thing at a time with parallel procesors, or (3) having a memory organization in which distinct ideas are stored not in a large number of distinct locations, but in distinct patterns of activity of a small number of locations (as with neural networks[1]). The remarkably fast response typical of an expert surgeon is thought to be possible because the human mind has both the second and the third of these features.

Figuring out a diagnosis involves not only the discovery of possible causes for the patient's symptoms, but also comparisons between the possibilities. The surgeon's first statement of the hypotheses already includes an implicit comparison between them: he identifies small bowel obstruction from adhesions as the first hypothesis but notes that external hernia is also a common cause of small bowel obstruction. This shows that the recognition of each hypothesis is not independent of the recognition of the other. Therefore, we cannot fairly characterize the surgeon's use of knowledge as the independent invocation of two rules, "crampy abdominal pain and history of previous operation suggest hypothesis of small bowel obstruction from adhesions" (common) and "crampy abdominal pain and external hernia (on physical exam) suggest hypothesis of small bowel obstruction due to external hernia" (uncommon but not rare). The expression of the relative strength of the hypotheses shows that the expert surgeon's use of his knowledge involves more than a simple process of pattern recognition. There is, at minimum, a comparison of the qualitative expressions of the hypotheses' relative frequency of occurrence.

Another way the surgeon's thought process supports the comparison between hypotheses is by identifying key information to look for. Thus, evidence that nausea and constipation are present or absent would support or undermine the hypothesis that the patient has amll bowel obstruction rather than gastroenteritis, flu, and so forth. This involves a focus on a metahypothesis that may be labeled "operation-needed." Information about the duration of the illness discriminates between the two hypothesized causes of small bowel obstruction. We see that the surgeon's first thoughts about the hypotheses carry witrh them an awareness of the bigger picture. These thoughts identify needed information because the surgeon usually seeks information at this juncture—in this case, information that can help to determine which of the two diagnoses is correct. Again, this is more complicated than a process of single-hypothesis recognition.

How can recognition be sensitive to context in these ways? The patterns recognized may be more complicated than simply "that looks like small bowel obstruction." The knowledge structure brought to mind may not be just a disease name, but a whole sequence of knowledge about what to do when you think someone has that disease. What is recognized, in this view, may be called a "script,"[2] an "illness script,"[3] or a "case description,"[4] rather than simply a category.[5] It includes what to expect and what to do in such a situation.

Such large knowledge structures, invoked by recognition, provide a flexible way of getting through familiar territory, yet at the same time they give a basis for handling unusual cases.[6,7] Problem solutions already may be contained within such a script. For example, when no obvious locus of obstruction was seen in the small bowel, the surgeon recognized the need to inspect its whole length thoroughly. The surgeon could have deduced this need using principles of logic, but he has probably already been through the prodcess many times. Thus the solution was recalled before he had time to think the problem through anew.[8]

Of interest, when a pattern does not quite fit, the doctor seems aware of this and directs more attention to the situation. For example, in the last paragraph of the transcript, he has an immediate recognition (pulmonary embolism) but exercises caution about it, either because it does not perfectly fit or because there may be danger in accepting the best-fit pattern. The surgeon can recognize quickly, but he can also recognize that quick recognition is not adequate.

The ability to recognize a decision in which one does not have 100% confidence is an important skill of the expert surgeon. In these cases, one needs to reflect, to review the raw data of the case by calling up the mental videotape of everything that has happened to the patient. The surgeon has learned to trust that "funny feeling" he gets when something is not quite right or a piece of hard data does not fit.[9]

In response to his reservations about the first qavailable pattern, the surgeon sketched out two other possible diagnoses. He then switched to thinking about what should be done immediately before gathering information for selecting among the diagnoses. He quickly decided on an action that would hedge his bets, protecting against the possible bad outcomes if any of the three hypotheses were true, yet doing no harm if any other of the three were true. Alghouth one cannot know this simply from reading the transcript, it is a well-learned response to a familiar situation, emphasizing the complexity and flexibility of an expert surgeon's knowledge and of the recognition process through which it is accessed.

1. Churchland PM: Cognitive activity in artificial neural networks. In Osherson DN, Smith EE (eds): Thinking: An Invitation to Cognitive Science, vol. 3. Cambridge, MA, MIT Press, 1990, pp 199–227.
2. Schank RC, Riesbeck CK: Inside Computer Understanding: Five Programs Plus Miniatures. Hillsdale, NJ, Erlbaum, 1981.
3. Schmidt HG, Norman GR, Boshuizen HPA: A cognitive perspective on medical expertise: Theory and implications. Acad Med 65:611–621, 1990.
4. Riesbeck CK, Schank RC: Inside Case-based Reasoning. Hillsdale, NJ, Erlbaum, 1989.
5. Abernathy CM, Hamm RM: Surgical Intuition. Philadelphia, PA, Hanley & Belfus, 1994, chapter 4.
6. Groen GJ, Patel VL: Medical problem-solving: Some questionable assumptions. MEd Educ 19:95–100, 1985.
7. Perkins DN, Salomon G: Are cognitive skills context-bound? Educ Res 18(1):16–25, 1989.
8. Salomon G, Perkins DN: Rocky roads to transfer: Rethinking mechanisms of a neglected phenomenon. Educ Psychol 24:113–142, 1989.
9. Abernathy CM, Hamm RM: Surgical Intuition. Philadelphia, PA, Hanley & Belfus, 1994, chapter 8.

20. BLEEDING DUODENAL ULCER

A 55-year-old man presents with gross melena. Four units of blood are required to restore his blood pressure to normal. Endoscopy demonstrates a posterior duodenal ulcer with an oozing vessel in the base. What are your thoughts?

If the duodenum is terribly scarred and you had to do a resection to get at it, I would insert a tube duodenostomy and close it. This procedure always works to keep you out of trouble in an emergency situation. ☐

On the fifth postoperative day the patient is jaundiced with a bilirubin of 8 and an alkaline phosphatase of 300; the other liver enzymes are normal. What would you do?

The patient needs endoscopic retrograde cholangiopancreatography (ERCP) or percutaneous transhepatic cholangiogram to make sure that I did not injure his common bile duct with my sutures. I would think back over exactly what I did, suturewise, at the operation and see if I feasibly could have put a suture around the common duct. ☑

On the seventh postoperative day, the patient vomits a large amount of blood. What would you do?

I would repeat endoscopy if at all possible. The patient could be bleeding from the suture line. I would keep in mind that the gastroenterologist can sometimes zap something and save the patient an operation. I would reoperate if they couldn't figure it out or if he was bleeding profusely. ☒

Surgical Observations

☐ Note that when a surgeon is given a very open-ended case like this (with minimal specific information), his thinking goes to a specific "get-out-of-trouble" technical trick (i.e., tube duodenostomy) before it goes to any other management thoughts. This is often how surgeons think; that is, they prethink the operation, using the worst-case scenario before they start. They figure out the 3 or 4 techniques they may need to get out of trouble.

☑ Once again, when faced with postoperative complication, the surgeon first thinks of what technical problems may have occurred in the operating room and what diagnostic studies may elucidate those problems. Specifically, he rewinds the videotape, back to the operating room, and visualizes exactly when and how he put in the sutures, did the anastomosis, ligated vessels, and so forth, and whether any of those specific procedures could have injured the common bile duct.

Observations continued on next page.

3 Similarly, the surgeon thinks of bleeding from the suture line (in this scenario without even knowing whether the duodenal ulcer is still in situ and has simply been suture-ligated or whether it was resected). The surgeon's first thought was the suture line. And his final statement is that if the bleeding is severe enough, no other diagnostic test or further work-up is needed except a return to the operating room. In other words, he has a trigger point for a patient who is unstable and/or bleeding profusely that takes him directly to the operating room.

Decision depends on recognition.

Cognitive Psychologist's Commentary:
Bleeding Duodenal Ulcer

The surgeon rapidly recognizes and responds to the situation. The elements of good decisions are present in these responses, although it is not easy to see them because the responses take place so quickly.

To make good decisions, one must know the options. In this think-aloud the surgeon comes up with appropriate options. If the situation were different, different options would come to mind. One of the features of the human memory is that ideas come to mind when they are likely to be needed.[1,2]

The surgeon must also know what can happen. Examples in the think-aloud include the surgeon's comment on the tube duodenostomy, that it can "keep you out of trouble," and his hypotheses about how he may have caused the postoperative jaundice by injuring the common bile duct with sutures.

A third aspect of careful thought about decisions is the awareness of how likely various events are. The more likely causes and effects come quickly to the surgeon's mind—e.g., the scarred duodenum, the bleeding from the suture line.

Decisions also must take into account how good or bad the results of one's actions can be. Such considerations are evident in this surgeon's script, as when he mentions the possibility of stemming the bleeding through the endoscope and thus saving the patient an operation.

A remarkable feature of surgeons' intuitive decision making is that it usually produces satisfactory decisions, although there is no explicit analysis to figure out which option is best. Experts' knowledge, of course, is at the center of their ability to make good decisions.[3] The elements of the decisions, listed above, are central categories in the expert's knowledge. The responses and recognitions in an expert's script, which are automatic now, have been built up over time. They incorporate the results of careful thought about each decision—not only the individual's thoughts, but also the results of analysis of what to do by the whole community of surgeons, communicated formally and informally in educational and professional settings.

1. Anderson JR, Milson R: Human memory: An adaptive perspective. Psychol Rev 96:703–719, 1989.
2. Abernathy CM, Hamm RM: Surgical Intuition. Philadelphia, PA, Hanley & Belfus, 1994, chapters 3 and 4.
3. Abernathy CM, Hamm RM: Surgical Intuition. Philadelphia, PA, Hanley & Belfus, 1994, chapter 7.

21. RIGHT LOWER QUADRANT PAIN

A 16-year-old girl reports right lower quadrant (RLQ) pain for 6 hours and mild RLQ tenderness. Temperature: 37°C. No nausea or vomiting. In midcycle of menstrual period. WBC: 7,800. No shift. What are your thoughts?

You are always worried about appendicitis, but it's early in the course of events. People usually don't have to worry about a ruptured appendix for 24–36 hours. If you don't think she has surgical indications, it's probably safe to watch her. It sounds like she probably has mittelschmerz because she is midcycle in her period (assuming she is not on birth control pills). She is very likely ovulating and experiencing pain from a little rupture in an ovarian cyst. You need to know if she is hungry or not, and if she typically has such pain during her cycle. You also need to do a pelvic exam, but it sounds like it might be mittelschmerz. I wouldn't operate on her at this point. ①

An ultrasound of the pelvis shows a slight amount of fluid in the cul-de-sac but is otherwise normal.

Same thing—she could have a ruptured cyst, and they didn't see it. Ultrasound would have been the next step. That's fine. ②

The pain persists overnight. Tenderness in the RLQ persists. Laparoscopy is performed. Tubes, ovaries, and appendix are normal. What would you do?

Appendix, tubes, and ovaries are normal. I probably would do a laparoscopic appendectomy while I was there, but I would not do anything further. Looking for a Meckel's with the laparoscopy would be the other possibility. It's the next morning, so you're not even 24 hours into the case. As far as you know, it's appendicitis, not a ruptured ovarian cyst—and no, it's not something surgical. I probably wouldn't do anything further at this point.

What triggers an operation for possible appendicitis? What does not trigger it?

I think the single most important thing is how tender the patient is over the appendix, in association with a compatible history. What does not trigger me to operate on appendicitis? Early in the course, less than 6 hours, less than 24 hours, I am not as worried. White blood cell counts don't help me very much. Patients who are hungry usually don't have appendicitis. A lot of people say they are hungry, but I think only once in my life have I had a patient with appendicitis who wanted to go to McDonald's for a Big Mac and fries, which is my standard question. They frequently say, "Sure, I'm hungry," and I say, "You want a Big Mac and fries at McDonald's?" and they go, "Uh, I don't think so." It's a rare patient who is hungry. I am inclined not to jump on them if it's particularly early in the course and the situation is confusing. But the single most important determining factor is how tender the patient is over the appendix. In a patient with localized tenderness and significant guarding who is over 24 hours out, I simply take out the appendix. It's a clinical decision. ③

Surgical Observations

1. The surgeon quickly synthesizes that it is "safe to watch her." The only other pieces of information on which he puts value are, "Is she hungry?" and "Has she typically had pain like this before?"

2. The surgeon thinks it's "fine" that an ultrasound was done, but it obviously isn't any help in his decision making. As with much lab and x-ray data, he's not opposed but knows they are unlikely to help.

3. This response is full of surgical pearls. Tenderness, length of time of symptoms, and anorexia appear strongly and in fact are essentially isolated as the only criteria for operation. They are presented not in sequential fashion but as three factors that are thought about in parallel, and given almost equal weight, although he notes that tenderness gets the edge in making the diagnosis.

Intuitive judgment decides the management of appendicitis.

Cognitive Psychologist's Commentary: Right Lower Quadrant Pain

This master surgeon's thoughts concerning whether to operate for suspected appendicitis are an example of intuitive judgment.[1] The surgeon pays attention to several factors simultaneously—amount and location of tenderness, duration of symptoms, appetite—and bases the decision on them. But he cannot verbalize precisely the rules governing the decision.

Judgments of this type have several features that differentiate them from knowledge in the form of rules.[2,3] First, the result of the judgment is one of three possible actions—send the patient home, wait and see what develops, or operate. Second, several features have a bearing on the judgment, such as patient's sex, age, and weight. Also relevant are features of the present illness, such as location, intensity, and quality of the right lower quadrant pain as well as the patient's appetite. But it is not just the current state of these variables that is important; the surgeon also pays attention to how they have varied over the past hours and days. These variables actually make the decision even simpler, for they allow the surgeon to focus on just two actions: send home versus wait or wait versus operate. Of course, as the situation changes, the surgeon may focus on a different pair of options, but at any one moment the decision is simply between two alternatives.

A third feature of such judgments is that the experts do not know exactly how they make them. They can say sensible things about each feature, such as "if the patient has an appetite, it is probably not appendicitis," but they cannot say how the various features are combined into their overall sense of whether they should operate.

This is not to say that the judgments are indescribable. If we had the luxury of watching the doctor encounter a large number of cases of right lower quadrant pain—cases that varied in factors such as age, sex, and weight of patient, description of pain (intensity, location, and history), and description of appetite (degree of loss and history)—we could produce a model of the doctor's judgment. The model would be able to predict the surgeon's judgments to a greater or lesser degree of accuracy.[4]

Such models usually have the following characteristics. If one of the features (e.g., degree of appetite) changes a *little* bit, it has a *small* impact on the decision to operate versus wait at a given time. If it changes a *lot*, it has a *large* impact. Second, you can compare the impacts of different features. For example, clear evidence of tenderness at McBurney's point is stronger evidence for appendicitis than lack of appetite. Third, the ways the specifics of the patient's presentation act together in the surgeon's judgment can be specified exactly in these models. Finally, people don't always make judgments consistently. These models can measure the degree of the expert surgeon's consistency or control in making judgments.[5]

Most expert judgments have not been studied in the manner just described. And, whether psychologists have studied the judgment or not, experts who make the judgments do not think about how they do it in terms of the model: relative weight, amount of control. They just know what they would do for each patient.

Presumably, master surgeons have learned how to respond to variations in right lower quadrant pain, learning from each other and from experience. The fact that it is hard for experts to explain the basis for their judgments raises the possibility that they don't understand each other as well as they think. For example, two expert surgeons may make their judgments using different models, although they think they do it on the same basis.[6] These questions have been explored for several types of medical judgment.[7,8]

1. Abernathy CM, Hamm RM: Surgical Intuition. Philadelphia, PA, Hanley & Belfus, 1994, chapter 8.
2. Buchanan BG, Shortliffe EH: Rule-Based Expert Systems: The MYCIN Experiments of the Stanford Heuristic Programming Project. Reading, MA, Addison-Wesley, 1984.
3. Abernathy CM, Hamm RM: Surgical Intuition. Philadelphia, PA, Hanley & Belfus, 1994, chapters 4 and 5.
4. Hammond KR, McClelland GH, Mumpower J: Human Judgment and Decision Making. New York, Praeger, 1980.
5. Hammond KR, Summers DA: Cognitive control. Psychol Rev 79:58–67, 1972.
6. Brehmer B: Social judgment theory and the analysis of interpersonal conflict. Psychol Bull 83:985–1003, 1976.
7. Wigton RS, Patil KD, Hoellerich VL: The effect of feedback in learning clinical diagnosis. J Med Educ 61:816–822, 1986.
8. Kirwan JR, Chaput de Saintonge DM, Joyce CRB, Currey HLF: Clinical judgment analysis: Practical application in rheumatoid arthritis. Br J Rheumatol 22(Suppl):18–23, 1983.

22. PELVIC FRACTURE

A 27-year-old man in a high-speed motor vehicle accident is brought into the ED. Evaluation shows a bilateral posterior pelvic fracture displaced 2 cm vertically. Cervical spine and chest x-rays are negative. Diagnostic peritoneal lavage (DPL) shows 90,000 red cells per high power field. Blood pressure: 100/80; pulse: 130. What would you do?

From the information you have given me, the patient has already had some work-up in the ED, although I am not sure whether the work-up has been in the sequence that I personally would have done. You made no mention of the basics—airway, circulation, whether the patient is breathing spontaneously. On the numbers you have given me, I am not inclined to act further other than to start some oxygen. I am worried about the fractured pelvis—it tends to bleed and by the time you've appreciated what's happened, it tends to collapse. I want two large-bore IVs. In an older person, I usually place a central line or a Swan-Ganz catheter as well, but in a 27-year-old man, two large-bore IVs will do for the time being.

The other thing is that, as a matter of routine, I would have the patient in military antishock trousers (MAST) and inflate them if necessary.

A count of 90,000 in the setting of a fractured pelvis is equivocal. In my situation, we would assess the rest of the injuries. As part of his radiology work-up, I need to know what the rest of his thoracic and lumbar spine are like.

Two hours later after 4 liters of lactated Ringer's solution, the hematocrit is 28. He has received 4 units of whole blood. His blood pressure is 110/70 and his pulse 140. Lumbar and thoracic spine films are normal. What would you do now?

I would also request a CT scan as part of the initial work-up, particularly in a patient with an equivocal lavage count—a CT scan of both the pelvis and the upper abdomen. Have we got results on that?

The CT scan shows a minimal amount of intraperitoneal fluid; otherwise, it is nondiagnostic.

From my point of view, I am prepared to pass the abdomen as normal. The count is not high enough. However, having said that, the amount of hematocrit and, more importantly, the amount of fluid required to maintain his blood pressure are high. Maybe there is higher-than-normal bleeding. □ From a fractured pelvis I would have expected something in the range of full blood volume in the first 24 hours. Two hours in, if it is needed, at least 3 units, 3 liters of crystalloid, 2 liters of whole blood. He has required a large amount of fluid. In this kind of patient, all else being equal, I would want the orthopedic department to consider very early fixation of the pelvis and restoration of normal ring integrity. You also have made no mention at all of the stage, whether he has neurologic deficit of his lower limbs.

The neurovascular exam of his lower extremities is normal. And now, 2 hours later, his blood pressure is 90/60. He's got 4 more units of blood, and his hematocrit is at 25. The fixator has been applied.

I would maintain fluids, and I am particularly going to look for evidence of ongoing bleeding, because he's still needing more than I would have expected in a patient like this once the fixator had been applied.

If on examination of the patient as a whole, I can find no other obvious source, very early on I would like to look at his aorta. I also would like another look at his belly, which with this volume of blood loss is likely to be distended but not obviously abnormal with this amount of pelvic or intraperitoneal bleeding. [2]

It is distended.

At this stage, I would consider an arteriogram of the pelvis, because if there is evidence of bleeding, it may be that we can see the source of the bleeding and perhaps embolize it.

Surgical Observations

[1] The surgeon is prepared to pass this abdomen as normal, despite the DPL, but then he immediately hedges. The hematocrit and the amount of fluid required to maintain blood pressure worry him because they are too high. We see that for the expert surgeon the hematocrit and the amount of fluid needed to maintain the blood pressure (particularly the latter, which is a poorly defined entity) have precedence over the actual red count level of the DPL, which would be the typical criterion governing what branch to take at that node in a formal algorithm.

[2] The surgeon mentions that abdominal distention is probably not going to be as helpful as it would have been if the patient had had the distention initially. Various signs and symptoms commonly change meanings as the case progresses.

The expert surgeon has several strategies for dealing with patients who don't fit specific categories.

Cognitive Psychologist's Commentary:
Pelvic Fracture

A simple description of experts' knowledge says it uses categories and rules.[1] Thus, the surgeon perceives the situation, labeling it as a category. And the surgeon knows what to do in each possible situation, has a rule that says in effect, "if it is such and such a category, do this action."[2,3] Experts have much knowledge in this form, which lets them recognize many situations, i.e., identify the appropriate category and respond to it. The algorithmic approach to clinical decision making requires this sort of knowledge: one must categorize in order to decide which branch to take at each node in a tree.[4,5]

A problem in any categorization scheme is what to do at the borders of the categories. Thus, what should the surgeon do when it is uncertain whether a DPL indicates abdominal bleeding? Or when the signs of shock are equivocal?

One solution is to write more rules to handle the uncertain cases. If other features are considered, the situation may no longer be on the borderline. This could be handled, for example, with a lexicographic procedure:

> Focus first on the most important diagnostic test. If the results are unequivocally high, operate; if they are unequivocally low, decide not to operate; if they are equivocal, look at the next most important test.

> If this second test is high, operate; if low, decide not to operate; if equivocal, look at the third most important test.

> And so on. . . .

The trauma surgeon shows such a strategy in deciding how to respond to the slightly elevated DPL. He doesn't decide to do a laparotomy, nor does he rule one out. Rather, he seeks additional information: how are the thoracic and lumbar spine?

A second strategy for dealing with a situation that doesn't fit well into a category is to think in terms of relations among multiple variables rather than in the yes/no terms of a category scheme.[6] Instead of identifying the patient's injury as exactly one category or another and doing the response appropriate to the category, an expert can identify the state of each of a number of variables and integrate them into a big picture, making a response that takes all the variables into account. The trauma surgeon seems to be thinking in this way when he says, "On the numbers you have given me, I am not inclined to act further other than to start some oxygen." Had any of the numbers varied enough in the direction indicating severe shock, the surgeon would have increased the aggressiveness of his resuscitation. Thus the response (degree of resuscitation) is a continuous function of multiple variables rather than a fixed response associated with a category identified as either present or absent.

A third possible response to categorical ambiguity is to make all the relevant responses—to consider that each of the pertinent categories is true and to make the appropriate response or at least to prepare to make it. This would involve paying attention to more than one possibility at the same time, mentally going down more than one path of the tree simultaneously. This is done most elegantly if one can make a single response that is appropriate for all possibilities, i.e., if one can hedge.

Human cognition tends to move from one idea to another, from one category to its competitor. Thus, the surgeon says first, "I am prepared to pass this abdomen as normal," and then flips to the opposite: "However, maybe there is higher-than-normal bleeding." Rather than to make a decision as to which hypothesis to accept, he prepares to act on both of them: for normal abdomen, do nothing special; for abdomen with pelvic blood, apply external fixation immediately; for abdomen that is on the borderline, "I would want the orthopedic department to consider very early fixation of his pelvis and restoration of normal ring integrity."

The surgeon is not committed to any of the cognitive psychologist's theories about how people always handle ambiguity. And it looks as if he will do any of them when needed—gather information about additional features of the situation and use it in a categorical manner; integrate information from multiple features into a noncategorical response; or prepare responses for more than one category simultaneously.

------

1. Abernathy CM, Hamm RM: Surgical Intuition. Philadelphia, PA, Hanley & Belfus, 1994, chapter 4.
2. Simon HA: What is an "explanation" of behavior? Psychol Sci 3:150–161, 1992.
3. Abernathy CM, Hamm RM: Surgical Intuition. Philadelphia, PA, Hanley & Belfus, 1994, chapter 5.
4. Eiseman B, Wotkyns RS: Surgical Decision Making. Philadelphia, W.B. Saunders, 1978.
5. Abernathy CM, Hamm RM: Surgical Intuition. Philadelphia, PA, Hanley & Belfus, 1994, chapter 1.
6. Abernathy CM, Hamm RM: Surgical Intuition. Philadelphia, PA, Hanley & Belfus, 1994, chapter 8.

23. VILLOUS ADENOMA OF RECTUM

A 65-year-old man is referred to you with a villous adenoma of the rectum located 6 cm from the anal verge and encompassing one-third to one-half of the circumference of the rectum. Biopsy shows "marked atypia." What would you do?

After either further colonoscopy or barium enema to make sure that the patient has no lesion other than the one described at 6 cm, I would take the patient to the operating room and, under general anesthesia, widely dilate his anus and lower rectal sphincters. Then I would actually remove the lesion transanally—and with good margins.

As sometimes happens in villous adenomas with large lesions, a central carcinoma may be found in the middle of the villous adenoma. If this proved to be true in the pathologic specimen, then further surgery may be required.

If there was actually an invasive carcinoma in the midportion of the lesion, I would return the patient to surgery, most likely for an abdominoperitoneal procedure on a lesion this low. [1]

Surgical Observation

[1] This is a perfect example of an experienced surgeon outlining the 3 or 4 basic considerations in a very succinct and concrete fashion. He makes sure that the patient has no other lesions; he believes that he can remove the lesion from below "with good margins"; he knows that the likelihood of a carcinoma is high; and he is prepared to do an abdominoperitoneal procedure if it is required. All of this is communicated in a nice flow of patient management from beginning to end.

The expert surgeon's response is characterized by its sureness.

Cognitive Psychologist's Commentary:
Villous Adenoma of Rectum

A major feature of this master surgeon's thinking about the hypothetical case is its sureness. Along with his recognition of the situation comes his choice of what to do, which is presented without hesitation and without consideration of alternatives.[1]

Of course the surgeon cannot predict what will happen—whether there will be a carcinoma in the center of the adenoma, for example. But for each anticipated possible event, he has a response clearly in mind.

One may question whether the surgeon's certainty brings with it a little rigidity, a reluctance to consider alternative approaches that may be better. Upon probing, of course, the surgeon knows very well the common alternatives and the arguments pro and con. Having considered them adequately in the past, he does not need to bring up an awareness of the controversy each time he faces the situation.

Exceptions can be seen in the master surgeons' thoughts about some of the other hypothetical patients. First is the problem of breast cancer, in which the patients demand that the pros and cons be reviewed for them. The disease affects many young women from the generation that has sought empowerment and self-determination, and because the need for treatment is not urgent (a matter of months rather than of days), they have time to question and inform themselves. Second are cases in which the expert surgeon has recently adopted a new procedure.[2] Here the controversy is fresh in the master surgeon's mind and ready to be shared. Third is the case in which the surgeon is involved in teaching residents and has acquired the habit of explaining (see think-aloud on Rectal Cancer, p. 95) or is very aware of the contrasts between the expert's efficient decision making and the slower, more deliberate thinking of the inexperienced surgeon (see the expert-novice think-aloud on Hemorrhagic Pancreatitis, p. 146).

---

1. Abernathy CM, Hamm RM: Surgical Intuition. Philadelphia, PA, Hanley & Belfus, 1994, chapter 2.
2. See discussion of inguinal hernia in Table 7.15 in Chapter 7 of Abernathy CM, Hamm RM: Surgical Intuition. Philadelphia, PA, Hanley & Belfus, 1994.

24. RECTAL CANCER

A 65-year-old man, referred by a family practitioner, has a biopsy-proved adenocarcinoma of the rectum, 8 cm above the anal verge. On rectal exam you feel the tumor at the end of your finger easily. The patient is in your office. What work-up would you use? What would you do?

I think it's important to review the slides. That's frequently forgotten. Then make sure that your pathologist agrees that there is cancer, because sometimes the original pathologist is wrong.

But let's say it's a clearcut cancer and you know it can't be anything else. Next you need to figure out the rest of the colon, either through a barium enema or colonoscopy. ☐ The gastrointestinal people would argue that they should do it and that colonoscopy is much more accurate than barium enemas. But good barium enemas are just about as accurate. You have to find out how good yours are. But if your institution is good at barium enemas, they're essentially as accurate as colonoscopy for lesions above 1 cm. Lesions below 1 cm are usually just excrescences that the gastroenterologist will frequently use to say, "See, we found something." But it will be a hyperplastic polyp; it won't be anything.

You find out how the proximal colon is and review the histology. Then you look at the patient and try to figure out if he will have the wherewithal to handle perhaps 6–8 bowel movements a day, from a coloanal anastomosis, early on. Is he willing to put up with the trouble that preserving his anus will entail. And if he is, then say, "Well, I think I can take your tumor out." This is a mobile tumor—right?

Yes.

You say, "Well, I can probably take out the tumor and save your anus, but it will cost you." And if he says, "Listen, just fix me up," then you say, "Okay, you're getting an abdominoperineal procedure," because he'd be profoundly unhappy that he was not brand new and had to put up with all the problems, like diarrhea.

He decides that he wants a coloanal anastomosis.

He doesn't want one of those bags. His aunt had it, and she was miserable.

Tell us how you prepare the patient for the coloanal anastomosis. Visualize and tell us how you would do the operation.

I'd get a complete blood count, a urinalysis, an electrocardiogram, and a chest x-ray. I really don't care about the last two, but they're needed for anesthesia. And I would get an operative permit.

Now you're in the operating room. There's no bowel preparation.

You can give him a bowel preparation. I'm not sure you need it, but we do it.

Visualize and tell us how you do the operation.

You open the abdomen. Then the next step is to look at the liver and feel the liver—feel it carefully because 80% of liver metastases are on the surface. There's another common occurrence in people—little liver cysts that feel hard. So if you feel something, then you have to look at it. You may need to extend your incision, but you're going to need a long incision from the xiphoid down toward near the pubis.

There are two reasons to figure out if he has liver metastases or to visualize the problem: (1) it will help postoperative planning for what to do next, and (2) it may influence what you do if you run into trouble deep in the pelvis. If he does have liver metastases, he's got a limited life expectancy, and you may not want to waste all the time that he has left in the operating room trying to get out his tumor. So the first thing to do is to evaluate the liver—and remember that a good exam is 80% accurate. So that takes care of the preoperative liver scan and all those other things.

The second step is to pick up the omentum, hold it up, and run your fingers down the aorta on either side. You just go "psssp," and if you feel little bumps, you consider the possibility of periaortic nodal spread. Periaortic nodal spread is basically as bad as liver metastases. The survival curve is the same.

The third point about liver metastases is how many and where. Does he have 1, 3, or 5? Are they localized? Is the metastasis easily resectable or is it not easily resectable?

Next I feel for a hiatal hernia, because a lot of older people who have never had trouble before will start vomiting after surgery and you don't know the exact cause. You don't know if it's a partial bowel obstruction or something else. And a lot of patients don't have their reflux manifest; it starts only postoperatively. Therefore, I like to check for a hiatal hernia so that sometimes I can explain why they don't seem to take food as fast as I like. Then check for other tumors—like a kidney tumor or a pancreatic tumor—and for aneurysms. You still haven't reached the pelvis yet. You want to evaluate the upper abdomen really well at this point. ② You may even want to feel for a second primary tumor elsewhere in the colon. It may have been missed.

The next step is to stick your hand down in the pelvis, behind the bladder. Don't mobilize anything. Just take your hand and push down. Try to feel the tumor. If you can't feel the tumor from above by palpation (at this point you should be close to the coccyx), you're going to have an easy dissection—and that's nice to know. And the tumor won't be fixed. Presumably you did a good preoperative exam and decided that the tumor was not fixed, but you want to check again at this point. In other words, you're trying to figure out what it's going to take to remove the tumor. And if you can't feel it or if it seems small, you can make plans. ③

If it's going to be easy down below, if you can't feel the tumor, and if the patient has one liver metastasis in the lateral segment, you say, "Why don't we take it out while we're here?" It's just a big liver biopsy. But if it's going to be a big deal in the pelvis, you leave the tumor in the lateral segment alone.

Now we're set up. You've decided about the upper abdomen, what you're going to do about it, the stage of disease. You know whether or not the disease is limited to the pelvis, whether or not the patient has a hiatal hernia (I wouldn't fix the hiatal hernia now, but it's nice to know about), whether or not the patient has a pancreatic mass, and so forth. The tumor is now completely staged clinically, and you're going to move ahead.

At this point, I take down the splenic flexure, if we're going that low into the pelvis. I don't worry about whether the sigmoid colon will reach—it probably won't. After taking down the splenic flexure, you divide the sigmoid colon at about the junction of the transverse and descending colon. The way to figure out where to divide the sigmoid colon is to pull it up and look for a line heading directly downward between the mesenteric fold and the mesentery. This line is the superior hemorrhoidal fold and the sigmoid artery. You follow it downward until you reach the left colic artery.

Some people argue that you shouldn't worry about the left colic artery or even try to save it. Just take the inferior mesenteric artery (IMA)—period. I can't argue with their point of view—take the IMA, live off the arcades. But divide the sigmoid colon at about that point. Divide it with a stapler. You can cover the end if you want.

Then you take the colon and start over—you literally start over. Take out your retractor. Push the colon up at the small bowel, and start over. You pack all of the colon out of the pelvis and out of the abdomen. And you prepare to do a radical hysterectomy. You're not going to do it, but you want the exposure you would get with a radical hysterectomy. And you pack the way a gynecologist would pack.

The next step is to find the ureters at the pelvic rim and to follow them down into the bladder. To do that, you have to cut the mesentery laterally on both sides. Then you pull up the bladder and find a plane between the seminal vesicles, which you usually can't see. But if you get the correct exposure, you can see a fusion plane right there. Take your scissors and cut across it a little bit. And after you open the perineal (Denovillier's fascia), take your hand, turn it around, and start pushing the bladder upward while you pull the rectum superiorly. Push up the bladder, and head toward the pubis, pushing it up. If you've done this correctly, you can get in a plane directly on the seminal vesicle in the male. Then you continue downward and find the prostate. Once you are past the prostate, you've gone far enough anteriorly from above. You hold the cut sigmoid colon taut as you can, you go about 5 mm past the sacral promontory, and you make a cut in the mesentery. You don't start on the sacral promontory because, if you do, you get into the sacral fascia and the surgical field becomes too bloody. Therefore, you go past the sacral promontory about 5 mm and then curve back. You open the mesentery a little closer to the rectum on that plane than you thought necessary. Then you start pushing the rectum forward with your hand—first with two, then three, then four fingers. Keep pushing it forward. You go down until you are past the coccyx. At that point you are in the perineum. If bleeding begins, you are in the wrong place.

Now you should be straight up anteriorly into the perineum and straight up posteriorly into the perineum. Next you pull the rectum laterally, with your fingers on either side of what I call the broad ligament. Both the broad ligament, which is between your fingers, and the rectum, which is held opposite, are free, and the ureter is lateral. Then you come down at a right angle, taking everything lateral below the ureter. And if you pull properly with your fingers, you'll see the middle hemorrhoidal vessels at the point where they come off the pelvic sidewall. You take them there with clamps.

Next the tumor is freed, and you continue downward in that plane until you see levators. (At this point I do something different: I turn the patient on his side.) You need to be 4–5 cm past the tumor. If you are not, and if you can see the levator, you cannot save the patient's anus. So you put his legs up and take it out. I've given up the lithotomy position, because I think it's more difficult than the transacral approach to the lower pelvis and perineum.

At that point, everything is freed, and you do a coloanal anastomosis. I tie a long sponge on the proximal colon and stick it in the pelvis behind the rectum. Then I take out the packs and close the abdomen with towel clips. I turn him on his side and take out the sacrum. Then I mobilize the segment into the wound and cut it off wherever needed. Then I grab the sponge and pull the colon down, sewing it to the anus under direct vision. Then I close the wound, put the patient on his back, and finish up above, because I like to close off the pelvis. Some surgeons do not, but I close off the pelvis. That's it.

Very good. But now I want you to assume that the patient came to you with the same lesion, but when you felt it with your finger, it was absolutely immobile.

In that case, you say to the patient, "We've got problems." Don't say, "You've got problems"—say, "We got problems." He'll want to know why. And the reason is simple: any degree of fixation means that the tumor is advanced locally. One, on that basis alone, he has severely limited survival. Two, he may be looking at two bags. He came in with a rectal tumor and never thought that he'd have one bag. Now you're raising the possibility of two—one for urine and one for stool.

An argument can be made that you can make the tumor mobile with preoperative therapy, either radiation combined with chemotherapy or radiation alone. This is true in about 40–50% of patients: whatever the cause of fixation, it will resolve with preoperative radiation. I think that it's probably worthwhile to consider this course, apart from anything else. When the patient wants to know when the operation is, you say, "Not right now." Then you start over. The first thing you do in terms of the pelvis is to send him to the oncologist for radiation therapy. Then you evaluate the rest of the colon and liver and all these other things. You are not going to operate on him. You order computed abdominal tomography, a barium enema, and a colonoscopy, all of which may change your approach considerably, because this patient has a much higher chance of liver and lung metastases or other disease than the first one. Assuming that he doesn't have any of these, you proceed with radiation and chemotherapy. So what happens after that?

The patient gets 6 weeks of preoperative radiation and chemotherapy. Then he's back in your office and wants to know when the operation is. You examine him again and find that the tumor size has shrunk to a degree that you think that there is a little mobility.

That's not good enough. The next step is an exam under anesthesia.

Under anesthesia you see that you can move the tumor in the pelvis.

So it's not fixed anymore. I'd approach it the same way we did for the other patient. Now we have a tumor that's mobile, and theoretically we can save his rectum.

During the operation you go down into the pelvis and find that the tumor actually is from lateral side wall to lateral side wall, absolutely packed in the pelvis.

That shouldn't happen. You shouldn't be surprised like that. That's part of the exam under anesthesia.

The exam under anesthesia shows that the tumor is fixed to the lateral pelvis, both sides.

The tumor is potentially resectable, both for cure and long-term palliation, but many people would consider the patient inoperable. He is inoperable with a standard abdominoperineal procedure, and anterior resection, or the operation I talked about before. That operation will cut through a tumor and leave him no better off than he was before the operation. Remember that the most actively growing part of the cancer is at the periphery; therefore, you're leaving behind the most actively growing part and taking out the dead tumor, which would probably sit there without doing much for a long time.

In this case you tell the patient that he has big problems. To remove the tumor will cost him his bladder, the lower half of his sacrum, and maybe a few other things. And he'll say, "That sounds terrible. I can't."

The next thing he will ask is "What happens if I don't do anything?" Essentially, you've told him that he's most likely to die of cancer, fairly indirectly but in strong terms, and that he has to rethink everything about what life is worth. If he doesn't have the operation, first he can look forward to the shutting off of his ureter, which may be present already. You may consider intravenous pyelography, but most of the time, at this point the patient has obstruction of the ureter and the tumor is probably invading his bladder. He'll tell you he had trouble emptying his bladder and that some crap is coming out, more than before. He's having trouble with his urinary stream from tumor invasion of his bladder, which is starting to shut off. That will be first.

The second thing to happen is that, while the radiation will hold the tumor in check for varying degrees of time, at some point the tumor will start bleeding again. And the bleeding will be very difficult to control because you can't embolize the vessels—too many are bleeding. He'll continue to bleed, and then he'll start to stink. So nobody will come to visit him.

And then the pain starts—the type of pain about which patients literally say, "If you can't do something to help the pain, I don't want to wake up. I'd rather die on the operating table than go on the way I am." It is a boring pain that you go to bed with and wake up with; it never goes away, and each day it gets worse. You hope to die, but you don't; the pain just goes on.

So he decides to have the operation. Briefly tell us the modifications you would make in the operation for a large pelvic-filling tumor.

The secret to removing the tumor is to cut the sacrum. Then it becomes rather easy.

You mean the sacrum above the tumor?

Yes. And the approach is lateral. In fact, going after the big tumor is what brought me to the transacral approach for small tumors.

How high can you take the sacrum?

From S3 down. You can actually go higher.

How do you manage the pelvic side walls when the tumor reaches from wall to wall?

You're outside the pelvic side walls when you come from below. You go up into the ischiorectal fascia and cut off the sacrum. At that point you've got levators coming down, but actually there's a thick band because the sacrum is cut. At that point, everything is freed from above. You take two big clamps, you go clunk, clunk— and it's out. It's easier than you think.

You're one-fourth of the way into this operation, and you encounter massive bleeding.

You don't encounter massive bleeding. I used to ligate the hypergastric arteries to prevent it.

Does that help?

No. I don't do that anymore, even though theoretically it helps.

Surgical Observations

1. The surgeon has a few routine items that he ticks off before actual patient management starts. A computer would be ideal at this stage, but it doesn't really get into the problem solving.

2. A very important point in exploring the abdomen is clearly and beautifully stated here. You should avoid going to the area of disease until you have explored the remainder of the abdomen and particularly thought about the implications of anything you might find and of other incidental findings. This is a time to think about the problem in general rather than to focus on the problem itself.

3. The surgeon makes a general statement about whether the primary tumor can be removed easily and talks about the implications of whether or not it's going to be easy. This sort of mental balancing act is very important in the management of the patient but very difficult to place into an algorithm or expert system.

The surgeon uses his hands to visualize the operation.

Cognitive Psychologist's Commentary:
Rectal Cancer

Although the reader can't see it, this surgeon thinks with his hands. He uses his hands as he explains the steps of the operation, indicating where anatomic features are as he imagines creating spaces and moving organs, showing the position his hands would take as he does maneuvers. When he says, "You hold the cut sigmoid as taut as you can, you go about 5 mm past the sacral promontory, and you make a cut in the mesentery," he moves his hands as if he is actually stretching and cutting the organ.[1]

His knowledge of the typical operation includes information in the visual, tactile, and kinesthetic modalities. His memory of individual operations would be in the same modalities, except that the particular details (if they were noticed) would be substituted for the generic details that he had in mind as he spoke here.

On this occasion the master surgeon thought aloud before a room full of about 15 medical students and residents. His gestures helped to communicate from his visualization of the operation to theirs. The students' ability to follow such an explanation depends on their familiarity with the anatomy and their experience doing or observing similar procedures. Often the teaching is done in the operating room, where the demonstration does not depend on the students' ability to generate visual imagery. But presumably the listeners are very knowledgable and can visualize along with him.

The ability to visualize is a fairly stable individual difference, although it can improve with practice, with the acquisition of knowledge, and with the discovery of strategies. Some students have difficulty following this sort of teaching, because they do not think easily with visual imagery. Although some people with poor imagery ability are excluded from medical school or figure out that surgery will be particularly difficult for them, a few who elect to train in surgery will never develop the visual sense to the degree they need.

The borrowing of techniques. This surgeon uses techniques that he recognizes as having originated with other specialties. For example, he packs near the colon the way a gynecologist would pack and goes in through the back the way a neurosurgeon would. These examples illustrate that techniques spread among disciplines.

---

1. Abernathy CM, Hamm RM: Surgical Intuition. Philadelphia, PA, Hanley & Belfus, 1994, chapter 10.

PART II

EXPERT/NOVICE THINK-ALOUDS

The same scheme for presentation of the cases is used as for the Master Surgeon Think-Alouds (see p. 1) except that the central or pivotal points in the thinking of the residents versus the attendings are highlighted in color.

25. Campfire Burn

26. Burn in Apartment Fire

27. Acute Carotid Dissection

28. Cerebral Vascular Accident

29. Thyroid Nodule

30. Pacemaker Complication

31. Solitary Pulmonary Nodule

32. Sepsis of Unknown Focus

33. Liver Laceration from Motor Vehicle Accident

34. Hemorrhagic Pancreatitis

35. Laparoscopic Cholecystectomy

36. Jaundice with Pain

37. Epigastric Pain

38. Abdominal Aortic Aneurysm

39. Left Lower Quadrant Pain

40. Small Bowel Obstruction

41. Pelvic Fracture

42. Rectal Bleeding

43. Acute Pain in Leg

25. CAMPFIRE BURN

A 12-year-old boy is brought into the ED after falling into a campfire and burning the extensor surface of his right forearm and the lateral surface of his right upper arm. How would you manage him?

3rd-Year Resident

This is a burn from a campfire, not a housefire. My concerns over complicating factors like smoke inhalation are a bit less. But there is still going to be local prevention and care as well as prevention of resuscitation problems. The depth and degree of the burn will make a difference—you want to make sure that he is hydrated. He probably has a deep burn and muscular damage. I want to **follow his electrolytes carefully** and to make sure that he is making a fair amount of urine.

In addition to local wound care—since he probably has cellular damage and may have compartmental damage with arm swelling—I want to keep an eye on the wound and even may consider **early fasciotomy** if there is swelling and hand dysfunction.

The other concern is to keep the wound clean. If this is an isolated burn that is not dirty and contaminated, then the objective is to create

Chief Resident

First of all, I would do a complete physical examination, including extent of the burn—whether it appears to be first-degree, second-degree, third-degree—and evaluate the distal pulses. Given his age and the fact that he has had injury to an extremity, he would be a candidate for **admission to the ICU**. At this point he really would not need significant fluid resuscitation, because it is probably less than a 9% burn. **He would need hydration and monitoring in the ICU.** [3]

He would need appropriate splinting to ensure adequate function of the extremity. He would need appropriate wound care, depending on the area of the wound. Regarding blisters, I would probably debride them. There is the possibility of an escharotomy—whether or not it would be necessary depends on clinical findings. Tetanus immunization may be appropriate, depending on his previous history, whether he has been immunized. I would not use prophylactic

Attending Surgeon

I assume that he is a healthy, young fellow with no preexisting medical conditions, no allergies, and so on. **The burn size is relatively small.** It is less than 9% because it falls only on one portion of the upper extremity. Therefore he would probably **need no fluid resuscitation** unless there is some other circumstance, such as extreme dehydration.

I would inspect the wound and try to make a judgment about its depth. Under ordinary circumstances, **he could be treated as an outpatient** with no risk of mortality. Since **it's not a circumferential burn,** [5] there is no problem with compartment syndrome. He probably doesn't need to be watched for that, but **you want to make sure that he has satisfactory distal circulation in his fingers.** [6]

I would instruct the parents to elevate the arm just slightly above the level of the heart to prevent excessive edema. I would dress the wound a protective barrier to prevent further infection and further loss of function. [1]

Determining the depth of the burn can be quite difficult because of the symptoms of a superficial burn, including pain. Deeper burns may be accompanied by loss of neuromuscular function, which I would assess and try to preserve. The swelling and tissue injury may cause further complications. [2]

The next day you are examining the boy's burn, and you're not quite certain what the depth of the burn is. But the depth determines what you do next. How do you determine the depth? Apply your assumption about depth to your continued management of the burn.

A partial-thickness burn, whether it be first-degree and related to the epidermis or involves the dermis, either superficially or deep, stands the best chance of retaining function. [4] If he has no evidence of a neurologic deficit, specifically sensory, and if the subdermal plexus is not invaded, the burn probably is related to the dermis alone. The patient probably has a chance of full recovery, because it's a second-degree burn. If he has no evidence of compromising joint spaces, I would treat him with localized wound care, specifically topical agents and splinting.

with silver sulfadiazine and have the patient return the next day. I always see the patient the next day and reinspect the wound. Then I try to make a decision about whether the wound will heal within 3 weeks. If the wound heals spontaneously within 3 weeks, the prognosis for the skin is excellent—good pliability, good protection, and virtually normal restoration of pigmentation. **If it appears that the wound will take longer than 3 weeks to heal, the patient should be advised that the burn should be chipped off surgically and skin-grafted, if possible.** [7]

antibiotics, and probably would stay with silver sulfadiazine as initial treatment of choice.

Two other points that I didn't mention. He should have tetanus immunization brought up to date. All these wounds are tetanus prone. He needs no prophylactic antibiotics. While inspecting the wound the next day, you want to make sure you haven't made a mistake assessing the patient and the condition of the wound. [8] Signs that would lead you to believe that it's a partial-thickness wound include maintenance of perfusion, **evidence of perfusion of the tissues, blisters, and erythema of the skin.** Erythema is thought to represent a first-degree burn, whereas **blistered skin is thought to be a second-degree burn.** On the other hand, if the blisters are desiccated and have a white waxy or discolored appearance, then the burn may be a little deeper. I would then indicate to the patient or the parents that the burn is a little deeper and may need to be operated on. [9]

Surgical Observations

3rd-Year Resident

[1] The resident is used to seeing large, severe burns and uses a mental list of *all* of the possible complications, such as compartment syndrome. In general, the resident overplays and overtreats the burn, assuming that it is deep ("into the muscle"), although no information is given in the presentation about depth. Experts do not have to do *everything*, as if *all* complications and diagnostic possibilities applied to the patient.

[2] The resident has no definite plan ("script") in mind for determining depth of burn. Again, the resident emphasizes *severe* muscular burn.

Chief Resident

[3] After following a clear script for burn evaluation, the resident still insists on immediate hydration, even after he notes that the patient "would not need fluid resuscitation." The resident is simply more comfortable with IVs and ICU.

[4] The resident knows principles of partial-thickness and full-thickness burns but fails to connect this concept to healing with or without grafting. Instead the resident uses a more vague term, such as "function."

Attending Surgeon

[5] The attending surgeon visualizes the burn while he is talking—it "only falls on one portion of the upper extremity" and is "not a circumferential burn."

[6] Unlike the resident, the attending surgeon has a simple rule for compartment syndrome: "watch distal circulation."

[7] The rules governing how he will decide whether or not to graft are simple and clear.

[8] The attending always challenges his initial diagnosis while moving ahead.

[9] The surgeon reviews his "script" for advising parents or patient regarding future course.

Inexperience leads to caution and conservative management.

Cognitive Psychologist's Commentary: Campfire Burn

The chief resident knows more about managing burns than the third-year resident. In fact, he mentions nearly every issue that the attending surgeon considers. But he is more cautious. For example, the attending surgeon would send the boy home and check him the next day, whereas the fifth-year chief resident would admit the patient to the ICU and possibly debride the blisters. The less experienced doctor, who has seen less and does not know what to expect, needs to keep the patient near and to be more actively involved.

The chief resident appreciates both sides of the issue. He knows the arguments that justify less caution, but he makes the cautious choice. This reflects, perhaps, his realistic assessment of his own knowledge: he knows that he can be surprised, that his prognoses are not fully reliable.

These think-alouds underscore the relation between ideas and behavior as expert knowledge develops. The fifth-year resident has developed the intellectual framework for considering all sides of the issues specific to treating burns. If asked, he could make the arguments for sending the boy home. But the options he chooses are more conservative. With several more years' experience, his behavior is likely to catch up with his ideas. This shows the importance of talking surgical philosophy, of hashing out the issues during the residency. Such discussions may not have immediate impact on the residents' behavior, but they lay the groundwork for the "wise" decisions later.[1]

Comment on the think-aloud method. The method of getting surgeons to think about "paper patients" is open-ended. The cases actually have relatively little specific clinical information. The surgeon must make assumptions to fill in the gaps and then take the problem from there. Two surgeons may be talking about different patients, and their responses, therefore, may diverge appropriately, revealing two alternative scripts pertinent to the case.

---

1. Abernathy CM, Hamm RM: Surgical Intuition. Philadelphia, PA, Hanley & Belfus, 1994, chapter 11.

26. BURN IN APARTMENT FIRE

A 47-year-old woman who is a smoker is brought in from an apartment fire with a 30% burn of the chest and abdomen. IVs are started, the burn is cleaned, and ABGs are drawn which show a PO_2 of 69, a PCO_2 of 25, and a carbon monoxide of 15. How would you manage the patient?

3rd-Year Resident

The first thing would be resuscitation. A 30% burn, so she will need **fluid resuscitation.** There are many different formulas—4 cc/kg per per-cent of burn area over the first 24 hours, with half of that in the first 8 hours. Then you go clinically. Start with a formula; if she is not making urine, if she remains in shock, give more fluid. If fluid is overloaded, you have to back off. Try to avoid the issue of crystalloid versus colloid. The next issue is her airway, because she sustained burns to her chest and abdomen. There was no mention of burns to her face, but it's quite possible that she would have an **airway injury.** She certainly has signif-icant carbon monoxide inhalation; she should be on 100% oxygen. Some people recommend hyperbaric treatments, but I don't believe that the carbon monoxide level is high enough to necessitate that. As for the burn, treatment is controversial. Some centers like to get the

Chief Resident

This is a fairly significant burn in a woman who is a smoker. ☐ Initially I would examine her and **assess the total percent burn,** which you say is 30%—just the chest and abdomen? I would assess her vital signs to see how she is doing. Assuming blood pressure greater than 100 and heart rate less than 110, I would commence with the physical exam, looking for singed eyebrows, singed nasal hairs, burned face. I would also start resuscitating her according to the Brooke formula—4 cc/kg per percent of the body surface area burned. Half of that is given over the first 8 hours and the second half over the next 16 hours. Also, because she was in a closed space, I'd perform a bronchoscopy to evaluate her airway passage. You say she had a carbon monoxide of 15, which is high compared with a normal level. If she has been a heavy smoker for a long time, that 15 may not be so elevated, but I would have to assume the worst

Attending Surgeon

Because she was burned in an apartment fire, she is at risk for an **inhalation injury.** And she should already have been started on the maximal amount of **nasal oxygen.** As part of the initial assessment, you go through the ABCs (airways, breathing, circulation), just as you would a trauma patient. The airway: if she is at risk for airway obstruction such as stridor, she should be intubated for airway protection. **If she has only hoarseness, eventually she may or may not need intubation.** Volume may indicate some degree of airway obstruction. If it's abnormal, I would inspect the airway. If it's not, I would just continue following ☐ the breathing, then the circulation, to make sure no emergency exists. She has more than just anterior torso burn ④; at any rate, she requires full resuscitation. One starts with a balanced salt and lactated Ringer's solution, using the formula to calculate an hourly dose. You multiply kilograms of body weight times the percent of body surface area burned. The first one-half of the calculation should be given the first 8 hours; you divide 8 into that number to get the hourly rate that you start with. You anticipate that if she has ventilation injury, she will require higher fluid replacement. **After you start fluid resuscitation, it becomes a clinical problem, and you throw the formula away.** [5] The patient should be treated on the basis first of **clinical response** and vital signs, then of perfusion, mental state, and urinary output, striving for about 60 ml/hour. **Initially wound care sort of takes a backseat,** [6] but when you get around to it, the wounds are generally cleansed and dressed, and silvadene is applied.

and go ahead and do a **bronchoscopy. If there was edema of proximal airways, I'd intubate her.** [2] I'd also give her a tetanus toxoid.

For treatment of the wounds, at this point I would use sterile dressings.

patient completely stabilized. Then, if it's a full-thickness burn, they do an excision and grafting at about 2 days. Others are more aggressive and recommend excision and grafting as soon as possible. If the burns are clearly demarcated, I'd go ahead with early grafting as long as the patient is resuscitated adequately.

Two hours after the patient is admitted, she is noted to have carbonaceous sputum. Physical examination reveals singed nasal hairs. Will these factors change your care?

You have to consider intubation if you're worried about a severe injury. She certainly can stand to be bronchoscoped. Depending on how the airway looked—**go ahead and intubate her** if she is maintaining good oxygenation and good ventilation. Clinically, it doesn't sound like she needs intubation. She could be bronchoscoped to examine the airway, or a scan could also demonstrate damage to the airway.

These factors go along with my initial assessment. I wouldn't wait 2 hours; I would find that out right away. And yes, it would alter things. I would proceed with **bronchoscopy.** Some people use ventilation scans. I would consider intubating her. The sputum itself wouldn't make me want to intubate.

No. [7] I would have suspected that these factors would confirm inhalation injury. **Whether she requires ventilation support depends on her clinical response.** And you would use the same criteria that are used to initiate ventilatory support in any patient. Ventilation scanning has been used in an effort to get a standardized technique for assessing inhalation injury. I would assume she had an inhalation injury. So we don't need a bronchoscopy.

Surgical Observations

Chief Resident

[1] Instead of the ABCs, the resident focuses on burn size, which the attending surgeon put as the last item of concern.

[2] The resident does not attribute the same morbidity and "down side" to intubation as the attending surgeon does.

Attending Surgeon

[3] The attending surgeon emphasizes "following the clinical course" and declines to make any hard and fast rules in the first part of his statement before he gets to the fluid resuscitation formula.

[4] The attending quickly checks the "30% burn" given versus his own mental assessment, realizing that it would take more than anterior chest and abdomen burn to give 30%.

[5] The attending surgeon emphasizes when *not* to use a formula or rule.

[6] The attending addresses the burn wound much later in his thoughts than the resident.

[7] Comfortable with his conviction, the attending cannot be talked into doing something just to "do something" or because it sounds "right."

The less experienced rely more on specific rules.

Cognitive Psychologist's Commentary: Burn in Apartment Fire

When presented with a "paper patient" burned on 30% of her body by a fire inside a closed room, the attending surgeon provides insight into a general issue in clinical reasoning: the proper place for rules or formulas. The formula in question concerns resuscitation. All three physicians considered fluid resuscitation appropriate, and each gave a formula for prescribing the temporal course of the resuscitation effort.

The least experienced physician spoke about this formula almost immediately—after only 15 words—as if this was one piece of information that he was sure of. He laid it out early while thinking in the back of his mind about what else he needed to do.

The chief resident, in contrast, started off with an overall reaction to the description: "This is a fairly significant burn." With more knowledge in a better developed script, he was able immediately to see the big picture. This provided an orientation for the plans he developed. He did not get around to presenting the formula for fluid resuscitation until after 70 words.

The attending surgeon also started with the big picture. His initial statment focused on the possibility of inhalation injury, which was not specifically mentioned in the description of the patient's symptoms. The others also considered this possibility, though later. The attending surgeon did not present the formula for fluid resuscitation until after 130 words. And soon afterward he commented, "After you start fluid resuscitation, it becomes a clinical problem, and you throw the formula away."

The hard knowledge—the memorable recipe for what to do in a situation—comes up earlier for physicians who know less and whose knowledge is less integrated and automatic. The more experienced physician wanted to grapple first with the whole situation, considering the important aspects of the case at a general level and getting oriented.

27. ACUTE CAROTID DISSECTION

The patient in the emergency department is a 44-year-old woman who was riding her 3-wheel all-terrain vehicle. She was wearing a helmet when she rolled the vehicle over. She was unconscious for about 5 minutes. She subsequently woke up, rode the ATV around for another 20–30 minutes, then rode back to camp. At the camp her level of consciousness began to decrease, and she actually passed out. At this point she was brought to the hospital.

3rd-Year Resident

This patient needs to be approached from the standard problem work-up. She has had an accident that could have resulted in multiple injuries. Clearly, you want to focus on her neurologic exam and her neurologic status. At the same time, you want to evaluate her ability to protect her airway and to ventilate; you want to ensure that she doesn't have an abdominal or chest injury that needs to be addressed. She probably would have the standard work-up, with standard laboratory tests, chest x-ray, cervical spine film, and peritoneal lavage. Then she needs CT scan to evaluate the head. During all of this you need to protect her cervical spine adequately, and she will probably need an endotracheal tube, which should be done nasotracheally because of the risk of cervical spine injury. What were the findings on her initial problem films? As you're getting her ready for the CT scan, you want to look carefully at the cervical spine to make sure that she doesn't have chest injury with hemopneumothorax. If her vital signs are stable, I would take her for the CT scan, with someone accompanying her. In the neurologic exam, obviously her level of consciousness is important, along with the presence or absence of localizing symptoms. The neurosurgeons should be made aware of her presence in the emergency department. A significant head injury with a lucid interval and then a rapid demise is the classic finding for epidural hematoma, although more probably a subdural hematoma, including contusion as well as some swelling, led to a decrease in the sensorium.

Attending Surgeon

A 44-year-old woman has had a head injury, and lucid interval, and then she passed out. First, I would want to check her ABCs and manage her airway. I would want to do a brief neurologic exam, focusing on her level of consciousness rather than on her reflexes and so on. **I would get a hematocrit to make sure that she had no hypovolemic problem and that in fact her injury is neurologic.** I would do a brief exam of her, start an IV, and look at her pupils.

After 30 minutes, all the initial work-up is complete. Cervical spine injury is ruled out, and the DPL is negative. Physical examination revealed decreased motion on the left side of her body. The patient was electively intubated and hyperventilated.

3rd-Year Resident	Attending Surgeon
(The resident was given the above and below information at the same time. The think-aloud begins below.)	I am becoming more and more sure that this is in fact a neurologic injury. You did not mention her pupillary response or whether there has been any change in her neurologic status. You might not have been able to see her for that long, but I am **certainly trying to find out exactly what speed is needed in terms of working her up** and potentially getting her to the OR, whatever needs to be done. You did not mention the vital signs, nor did I. I should have asked for the vital signs or any changes in them. It is a left-sided lateralizing sign. I would assess how long she has been in the ED and whether there have been any changes to see if I had time to proceed to the CT scan. Almost invariably, I would have enough time. I would proceed to the CT scan.

The patient was taken for a CT scan of the head, which showed no evidence of contusion; in fact, the scan was quite unremarkable.

The patient has lateral findings, with a CT scan that shows no clearcut lateral lesion. ① She may have a contusion that just is not apparent. She should probably be treated for brain swelling with hyperventilation, minimal fluids, careful observation, and head elevation. Depending on what her ventricles look like, I may want to consider a **ventricular pressure monitor.** In a patient with lateralizing findings and an unremarkable CT scan, you want to consider other possibilities, such as carotid dissection. I think the next step in her work-up probably would be an angiogram. ②

Now that we quickly resolved that issue, **we have to think about the other causes of neurologic injuries that are a little more subtle.** Because she is already in the imaging department and I see normal CT scans, ① with no evidence of brain injury, **we have to think about an arteriogram**. I suppose we have to think about other spinal injuries. In any case, we have to continue down the differential diagnosis of where this lesion may be coming from. I think that the next step—assuming that her vital signs are stable and that nothing else is showing up—is an arteriogram.

A carotid angiogram was done and revealed a carotid dissection.

Was the vessel intact? The literature is controversial about the best method of managing acute carotid dissections. Some people would elect to heparinize, and a great deal of literature suggests that immediate surgery is also appropriate.

I would want to know what that flap on the arteriogram really means—whether it was occlusive or just a little defect and whether the carotid artery was flowing. It probably was, if you saw the flap. It is certainly a lesion of great liability, and within 2 or 3 hours—a reasonable time if we have been really thorough on the work-up—I would take her immediately to the OR. ③

Surgical Observations

[1] Note that both surgeons repeat the significant history at this point.

Resident

[2] The resident, as he was talking, suddenly realized that with this combination of information (i.e., hemiparesis with a normal CT scan) a carotid dissection was a possibility. This type of insight often happens as you are describing a case to a colleague and thinking aloud about it.

Attending Surgeon

[3] The attending surgeon, realizing that a tough decision is about to be made, wants to know detailed information about the arteriogram, which is going to direct the patient's care. He really wants to see that arteriogram. Thus, the simple algorithm below is inadequate:

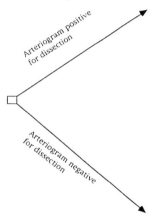

Instead, the spectrum of arteriographic findings has to be weighed simultaneously with many other features of the patient, such as current status of hemiparesis, general health, and time since neurologic deficit.

The net of knowledge covers all cases.

Cognitive Psychologist's Commentary:
Acute Carotid Dissection

In the acquisition of surgical knowledge there is a movement from the general to the specific. This is evident at several points when the resident knows the big picture but cannot move in and deal with the situation in detail.

For example, when carotid dissection was discovered on the angiogram, the resident's response came from "the top," the most general level: "The literature is controversial about the best method of managing acute carotid dissections." This general knowledge includes the major options: heparinization versus immediate surgery. But it does not include a well-integrated, quickly available sense of the factors that control that decision—the factors on which the literature agrees or disagrees. For the resident, the controversy is external rather than internal. The resident knows that surgeons argue about the best method of management, and if given time to ponder, he or she could probably recall some of the central factors in those arguments. But this knowledge is not yet the resident's own; the resident does not have an internal model of what factors favor heparinization or require surgery.

The expert surgeon, in contrast, knows the problem "internally," intimately, intuitively. The expert wants to see more of the angiogram, because he knows how to interpret what he sees in terms of his general understanding. He knows what questions to ask and what to do with whatever answers are given.

The resident, of course, is "on the way"—expert knowledge is in the process of development. Thus when he or she recognized the problem—the anomaly of lateralized symptoms with a normal CT—the resident knew what to do in terms of treatment and looking for other possible causes.

In another example, after hearing the first description of the case the resident acknowledged the many aspects of responsible care—awareness of the danger of head injury, assurance that the patient can breathe, sending a heads-up to the neurosurgeons. The expert is more focused: neurologic injury is a high probability, a potential hypovolemic problem needs to be ruled out, and a central question is what speed is required. The differences are a question of fine tuning; the resident knows the details but takes longer to get to them.[1]

In general, the knowledge that the resident is acquiring, after a few years, is like a net—it covers everything. Initially the mesh is big in any particular area, but with experience the knit becomes finer and finer. The density of knowledge is uneven, with different areas of the net knotted tightly or sparsely depending on individual experience. But everything is covered by the net, so that one has a response to anything that comes up, even if the response is very general, such as "Well, I know there is controversy about whether to heparinize or operate." This means that there is always something to connect new knowledge to.

In contrast, the raw novices in clerkships and internships have vast gaps in their knowledge; they lack even a general orientation to the cases they observe. It is not until the resident's net of knowledge has come to "cover everything," even if only sparsely, and to cover certain things quite well, that he or she begins to feel overconfident.

---

1. Abernathy CM, Hamm RM: Surgical Intuition. Philadelphia, PA, Hanley & Belfus, 1994, chapter 4.

28. CEREBRAL VASCULAR ACCIDENT

A 65-year-old woman presents with a 2-week history of weakness in the right hand and leg. What would you do?

2rd-Year Resident

I would do a complete exam to see if anything else is obvious. Are there any other cranial nerve defects? Is anything else in her neurologic exam missing.

What else would you do?

After completing the exam, I would find out if she has any risks for stroke, artery disease in her neck, or heart disease. I would make sure she doesn't have diabetes. That's it.

Chief Resident

First, I would get a history and physical exam. I'd assess whether any associated neurologic changes suggest a stroke, a stroke in evolution, or an impending stroke, such as TIAs. Has this been a continuous process, or did the symptoms suddenly appear?

I'd get a CT scan of her head as well. I would work up her carotid arteries, first with duplex ultrasound, then with CT scan. I would proceed on the basis of those findings. I also would do a complete vascular examination, looking for other potential vascular problems. I've found by experience that people with one vascular problem in one area often have vascular problems in other areas. I'd also feel her aorta, check her distal pulses, and so forth. In addition, I'd look at her **history for possible cardiac problems.**

Attending Surgeon

History and physical wise, I would want to know if she had ever had any episodes like that before, or any other neurologic events, or any other indication of **arrhythmia** or atherosclerotic problems. If she was clean from that aspect, I would probably order a CT scan of her head—presuming there are no other tricks to the neurologic exam—just to exclude tumor or subdural or other space-occupying lesions. Once I was satisfied with that, I would probably run her by the noninvasive lab, but regardless of those results, she would probably get an **arteriogram.** □

Duplex ultrasound reveals a high-grade stenosis of the left internal carotid artery (ICA) and an occlusion of the right ICA. Carotid arteriography demonstrates an occlusion of the right ICA and 95% stenosis of the left ICA with an irregular plaque. What would you do?

Because of the patient's recent history, I have to state again that I'd get a CT scan to look for evidence of a

She has been improving over these 2 weeks? What would I do? I would find out if she has

I would counsel her that she's at **extremely high risk for further events and that they will**

coronary artery disease. She's symptomatic from an injury, from a low-flow state because she doesn't have any symptoms on the other side. I think you're going to have to try an endarterectomy.

recent stroke. That would make a significant difference in terms of the staging, the specific timing of operative intervention. If there is no evidence of a recent stroke, I would proceed with addressing the plaque, the stenosis.

Wait a second! Her symptoms are right-sided, and it's a left-sided stenosis. So **I shunt her, regardless of the stump pressures.**

be potentially catastrophic. I would review in my mind the options, such as an external carotid-internal carotid (EC-IC) bypass, which is out of favor but in situations like this it's a thought. [2] I would reject that option and fix her left carotid artery. Using general anesthesia and a shunt, I would do a left carotid endarterectomy.

The patient was admitted to the hospital. A CT scan of the head demonstrated a small subacute infarct of the left cerebral hemisphere. She was treated with IV heparin and admitted to the ICU. Her neurologic symptoms partially resolved over the next 12 hours. Now what would you do?

You can continue to treat with heparin and see if resolution continues, but you have to solve the problem. At some point you still have to go into her carotid.

In that case—(pause)—these symptoms have been going on for 2 weeks—(pause)—I would forego an operation at this point, with demonstration of a recent infarct. I would forego an operation and assume that her symptoms are secondary to the stroke, not due to an ongoing decreased blood supply or embolic plaque upstream. I would continue to treat her with heparin and do the operation in approximately **8 weeks' time.** [3]

This addresses one point that I didn't address—the timing of the left carotid endarterectomy. If the CT scan reveals an infarct, which is unusual, I would try to get specific information from the CT scan or from MRI about the acuteness. These studies may be able to tell you that, depending on the amount of edema around that infarct. But I think that the patient is in great danger. **I would not worry about converting the white infarct to a red infarct;** she's 2 weeks past the initial event and she has improved. **Sometime in the next week** or two after I have given her aspirin and so forth, **I would fix the carotid artery.**

Comments from the surgeon who presented the case:

This is a real case, and we decided to operate on the patient acutely. In our way of thinking, the infarct was small on CT and the patient had a partial hemiparesis that was resolving, but she had such a high-risk lesion that to wait 6 weeks, we thought, would expose her to a stroke risk of approximately 20%, whereas to operate acutely would expose her to an approximately 10% stroke rate, perhaps less. We chose to cut her relative risk.

Surgical Observations

Attending Surgeon

[1] The attending surgeon knew what the struggle was going to be and pressed hard for any subtle clue, such as edema on the MRI or CT. He was trying to get a feel for how acute and how fresh the stroke was, for how fragile the brain was. You may be able to get some clue from the CT or MRI.

[2] The attending surgeon thought about an unproven alternative, the EC/IC bypass, which he notes is out of favor. He needed to do something fairly benign, even though it has not been proved of benefit in controlled clinical trials. However, the patient is not a controlled trial; that is, in her extremely high-risk situation she may benefit from an EC-IC bypass in a way that not all patients in the controlled trial would benefit. He is dancing around because he doesn't have many options to get the patient past this hurdle without stroke.

Chief Resident

[3] Heparin is not advisable in this patient. It involves a risk of bleeding that you do not need to take.

Deciding how long to wait before operating involves thinking with rules of thumb, with analysis, or with intuition.

Cognitive Psychologist's Commentary: Cerebral Vascular Accident

The surgeons' thoughts about this case reveal several aspects of surgical intuition[1] that are related to the question of how long to wait before operating.

The second-year resident had a common-sense response to the case, a quick intuitive take that she could not follow through on because of lack of knowledge. For example, the resident knew that operating on the carotid artery would be necessary "at some point," which shows that she grasped the general picture—she knew what was most important, but she was not confident enough to speak of the details.

The timing of the operation. The timing of the carotid endarterectomy was key in this case. The attending surgeon has identified the ultimate struggle between the studies in the literature that show patients to be worse off with early surgery, versus the high chance of stroke for every week that nothing is done.

As the surgeon who presented the case explained, the patient was actually operated on at the time (second day in hospital) rather than waiting. This violated the standard practice that after a recent stroke one should wait before operating on the carotids in order to avoid "turning a white infarct red." He had done the operation early after careful consideration and reading, figuring that although the probability of intraoperative disaster was 10%, the probability of an equivalent disaster during a wait of several weeks was 20%.

The chief resident, following the standard cautious practice, said that he would wait 8 weeks on top of the 2 weeks the patient had already waited before coming to the hospital. The attending said he would wait another 1 or 2 weeks, which would lessen the time during which a disaster could happen. This is an example of the master surgeon's intuitive judgment: without explicitly analyzing the situation, he came up with a delay period that reflects the various factors—balancing the danger of "turning the white infarct red" by operating immediately against the danger that another white infarct may happen during the delay. Typical of the processes usually involved in judgment,[2] his immediate intuitive response represents an average of the conflicting considerations: he chose to wait a short period, a compromise between waiting a long period and not waiting at all. His thinking on this issue was an intuitive, integrative judgment rather than the result of a simple rule (like the chief resident) or a careful analysis (like the surgeon who presented the problem).

---

1. Abernathy CM, Hamm RM: Surgical Intuition. Philadelphia, PA, Hanley & Belfus, 1994, chapter 2.
2. Abernathy CM, Hamm RM: Surgical Intuition. Philadelphia, PA, Hanley & Belfus, 1994, chapter 8.

29. THYROID NODULE

A 31-year-old woman has a 3-cm mass in the left lobe of her thyroid gland. Fine-needle aspiration shows thyroid follicular cells with some atypia. What would you do?

3rd-Year Resident

The presence of atypical cells has some bearing on the management. However, a nodule in the thyroid lobe may be **malignant or benign** (you cannot tell based on aspiration cytology in this case). Are you interested in my initial management?

Yes.

Do I like the feel of the family history? I want to know if she has any associated problems in her family, things like that. Is the mass hard? On thyroid scan, is it a hot or cold nodule? Those are important points to establish. Does she have normal thyroid function? Is she hyper- or hypothyroid?

Does any of that make a difference?

With what I would do ultimately? Not really. I would like to see if she has any palpable adenopathy, but basically this patient is going to need surgery. I would entertain doing a **subtotal thyroidectomy** as an initial procedure. You cannot tell whether this is a malignancy on the basis of fine-needle aspiration. If it were a malignancy and you do a subtotal thyroidectomy, you have to entertain the possibility of going back, reoperating, and taking out the opposite side. ☐

What do you mean by subtotal?

With a subtotal I would do a lobe and isthmus and a partial thyroidectomy on the opposite side, most likely preserving part of the upper lobe.

Attending Surgeon

I would be concerned that she has a thyroid carcinoma. Did she have a thyroid scan? ☐

No scan.

No scan. I may obtain the scan to determine whether the nodule is hot or cold. It is not particularly going to make a difference in what I do. Obviously, I would do a thorough history and a thorough physical. Is there any relevant family history? I would pay attention to other systems to see if she has any other endocrine problems. It is going to come down to doing a neck exploration, and I would do a **subtotal thyroidectomy.**

What do you mean by subtotal thyroidectomy?

I would remove the entire left side, looking for and trying to preserve the parathyroid, if possible. I also would take the isthmus. And on the opposite, the right side, I would try to leave a 5-g rim of tissue based on the inferior thyroid artery to preserve the parathyroid.

After a thyroid lobectomy and isthmectomy, during which the frozen section is returned as benign, the patient awakens and is noted to have laryngeal nerve palsy. What would you do?

This is postoperative—the patient is out of the operating room, extubated, and in the recovery room or ICU. If you have absolutely no indication during surgery of whether or not you have injured the nerve. . . . During the operation, was the nerve adequately identified? No clues like that? **If you feel you may have merely created a traction injury, it may resolve.** A lot of effort needs to be made at the time of surgery to see whether or not you

Did I examine the laryngeal nerve? I would have examined the cords on the way out. And there is laryngeal nerve palsy? **There is not a whole lot that I can do at that point.** I do not think there is anything I can do surgically to correct the laryngeal nerve palsy. I would wait to see what the

3rd-Year Resident *(Cont'd.)*

can identify the nerve and try to protect it. If you feel you have done that, it may very well be a traction injury that may resolve.

Attending Surgeon *(Cont'd.)*

permanent pathology sections show and whether the palsy is permanent. [5]

On the third postoperative day, the permanent sections return as follicular cancer. What would you do?

This is a patient in whom you have done a lobe and isthmus. You see that you have cancer plus laryngeal nerve injury.

The cancer has been inadequately treated surgically. There is too much residual gland in the remaining lobe to ablate with radioactive iodine. You are going to have to go back into the other side. With a patient who has a contralateral nerve injury that may be permanent, you have the possibility of causing airway obstruction if you injure the nerve on the opposite side. But this patient needs an essentially **complete thyroidectomy** to treat her thyroid cancer. [2]

The whole gland?

You could do a subtotal thyroidectomy and leave a small portion of tissue because that can be ablated with radioactive iodine, but I think you would try to remove as much of the gland as possible on the other side and take great caution to preserve not only the nerve but the parathyroid tissue.

Other questions are important, but they are not going to keep me out of the neck. [3]

You need to know whether you have paralyzed the vocal cords before surgery.

I would never be in this position to start with. I already have done the operation. At this point, with the follicular cancer, obviously I would counsel the patient very closely about possible injury to the laryngeal nerve on the other side since a clumsy oaf had cut it on one side. And I'd go back and do a **total thyroidectomy with careful sparing of the nerve on the other side.**

Surgical Observations

3rd-Year Resident

[1] The resident hedges on almost everything. He knows that a subtotal thyroidectomy is appropriate in this setting but hedges by saying "initial procedure." Once he says that, he reviews in his own mind that he cannot be sure if the nodule is malignant on the basis of cytology. He also seems to be a bit confused about whether the subtotal procedure is adequate for certain types of thyroid malignancy.

[2] A good grasp of the considerations is evident. But the resident does not want to weigh the morbidity of returning to the OR for completion of the thyroidectomy in the patient with a laryngeal nerve palsy versus the inadequacy of the treatment of the thyroid cancer. He doesn't seem to match the two clearly against each other.

[3] Now the resident has become bolder in his thinking and decided that nothing will keep him from going back to remove the remaining gland. Considerations include the following: (1) you need to know if the cord is definitely paralyzed before going back into the neck. (2) You need to know if you identified the

Continued on following page.

nerve—how comfortable are you when reviewing the videotape of the surgery in your mind that you did not cut the nerve, that you identified it and kept it out of harm's way? In other words, how certain are you that the problem is a traction injury? (3) If indeed the cord was paralyzed and the nerve was permanently injured, not many surgeons would go back into the neck for residual tissue. They would manage with what they had.

Attending Surgeon

4 The attending does a nice job of addressing the central issue of concern—whether or not a thyroid cancer is present. He then quickly asks a question, perhaps so that he can gather his thoughts—or perhaps the question helps him to focus his thoughts.

5 The attending does a sound job with questions regarding the laryngeal nerve injury, particularly whether or not he examined the laryngeal nerve at the operation (the mental videotape review). It is interesting that the attending also anticipates that the pathology report may pose a problem.

Another attending surgeon comments:

When I awaken the patient, I immediately ask the anesthesiologist to check whether the cord moves. If the cords don't move, some people talk about going back to take a look immediately. **If you attempt to identify the nerve every time, the decisions are easier.** Do we do thyroidectomy without identifying the nerve? Yes. Occasionally you cannot find the darn nerve, and you say, "Well, the darn thing is out of the way. Let us just stay right on the gland." Then you are tense. If the patient wakes up with vocal cord paralysis, you are stuck. You just have to watch and wait. Now, you mentioned that you would leave the superior pole on the right side. If you took the inferior pole, you can devascularize the front parathyroids on the right side.

Correct plans before executing them: exercise caution.

Cognitive Psychologist's Commentary: Thyroid Nodule

The third-year resident shows hesitancy and is reluctant to commit himself to a specific procedure. This contrasts with the sureness of master surgeons in a number of the previous think-alouds (e.g., Villous Adenoma of the Rectum, p. 93) as well as with the attending here.

Tentativeness about one's proposed actions is a reasonable strategy at a middle stage of experience. One knows enough to recognize the general situation, yet one is surprised frequently enough that one wants to hang back a bit. The plan that comes to mind may not be correct, and caution allows it to be corrected if it is wrong or incomplete before any damage is done. There are three potential sources of correction:[1]

1. One can correct oneself, recognizing errors or gaps as one reviews the plan. Stating it aloud puts it out, so one can look at it (see also the chief resident's think-aloud on Jaundice with Pain, p. 152). The thinking of intermediate surgeons puts a larger burden on working memory than does the thinking of experts;[2] thus they need to adopt an approach that allows them (1) to take longer, allowing their minds to work, and (2) to hold up tentative decisions for review, because the plans otherwise would decay out of short-term memory. The "hesitant" style of thinking serves both functions.

2. The people with whom one is talking can correct the plan. Where the first-year resident may wait for others to tell him or her what to do, the third-year resident knows more and can produce the plan for others to review. As he or she gets better, others make fewer and fewer corrections. This provides a gauge for both the resident and his or her colleagues about the resident's progress.

3. The situation can provide the corrections. One goes into the actual situation tentatively—operating slowly, thinking at each step, or discussing it with the others. One sees aspects that one did not anticipate during planning. Although one knows how to respond to these aspects when they actually arise, one does not know the situation well enough to anticipate them ahead of time. At a certain stage, one can rely on oneself to know how to recognize situations when one sees them, just as one can rely on oneself to be able to recall the details of the operation after the fact.

At this stage in the development of his expertise, the third-year resident knows the dimensions of the situation, but is not "well calibrated"; that is, he knows what is traded off against what but does not know the exact exchange rate. His scripts are not sufficiently refined; he needs to look very carefully as he moves.

This particular case highlights the need for caution. In thyroid operations, one needs to identify and to protect the laryngeal nerve during the operation. One must know ahead of time to do this, not wait for feedback—whoops, the patient will always be hoarse! The attending considered it automatic to have done that, and mentioned only the steps he would take to protect the parathyroid.

Hedging, or being hesitant, is a strategy for dealing with the risk of error. The basic tradeoff is between quick action that risks an error and slower action with the possibility of discovering and correcting the error. The costs of the slower approach are that it takes more time (which is money) and the possibility exists that patients may die in emergencies when quick action is needed. The costs of acting confident are that more errors might be made and one may miss the opportunity to learn. As one gains experience, there is less chance of error if one acts fast; thus there is a natural shift toward speed rather than caution.

Caution also has social costs, for one looks less "expert" when one hesitates. Caution that is appropriate at one stage—say the third year of residency—may be viewed as inappropriate at the fifth year, a sign that one has not developed as rapidly as expected. Conversely, confidence that accompanies good surgical results is admired, but confidence that leads repeatedly to disaster invites negative assessments of one's character as well as one's surgical ability. The degree of caution in a surgeon's thinking, therefore, is a matter both of how much the surgeon knows and of general personal choice or personality. Some surgeons are more risk-taking or confident than others.

---

1. Abernathy CM, Hamm RM: Surgical Intuition. Philadelphia, PA, Hanley & Belfus, 1994, chapter 11.
2. Abernathy CM, Hamm RM: Surgical Intuition. Philadelphia, PA, Hanley & Belfus, 1994, chapter 4.

30. PACEMAKER COMPLICATION

You are in the OR and you have begun to put a ventricular single-lead pacemaker in a 79-year-old woman using the subclavian approach. She is awake on the operating table, and the anesthesiologist is monitoring her. You have inserted a needle twice and have gotten nothing back. On the third attempt, the syringe is filled with what appears to you to be arterial blood. What do you do?

1st-Year Resident	3rd-Year Resident	Attending Surgeon
I withdraw the needle and apply pressure for about 10 minutes. Then I attempt to reinsert the cannula. **Same side?** Yes. [1]	The natural thing to do is just to pull out and put pressure on the area. With the subclavian approach you are **not going to be able to put adequate pressure** on some patients' arteries. [4]	I am **worried about her hemodynamic status.** Initially I would want to make sure that she is **ventilating** adequately. I then make sure that she is not bleeding into her chest. At this point, I'd like to look at her, to make sure she is ventilating effectively on both sides and that her heart rate and blood pressure haven't changed. Her brain is a reasonably good way of assessing how well she is perfusing—whether she is thinking, able to talk. I ask her a question, and she responds. As a first step, I use her mental state to assess her airway, breathing, and circulation. I am most worried about invisible bleeding in her chest, so I use her heart rate and blood pressure as a monitor of that. I still have the needle in her subclavian space. If the needle is 20 gauge or smaller and if arterial blood is coming back, I would be comfortable pulling the needle out and seeing what happens. [7]

You make one more pass. This time you're successful and you get into the vein. You insert a sheath and start the lead for the pacemaker. You note that the lead appears to be in the apex of the right ventricle. The anesthesiologist reports that the pressure is 60/palp with a sinus rhythm.

I make sure that she is in a sinus rhythm and rule	60/palp, normal sinus rhythm, trouble getting	60/palp. I guess I would still do the same thing again. I want to make sure she is ventilating adequately, that she is moving air effectively. I am obviously worried that she is now losing

out hypoxia. I send for stat hematocrit and look at the left subclavian area for hematoma. [2]

volume into the side that I am on, the left side, so I would check her for airway and ventilation to make sure she is moving air on both sides.

I assume that she is **tachycardic at the same time.** If she is, it confirms my impression that she is losing volume into her right chest. If she is not, I am willing to assume that she doesn't need to have associated tachycardia, and I still think she may very well be losing volume in the right chest.

The other possibility, of course, is that I could have **perforated her heart.** I would think that is vanishingly **unlikely** [8] with a soft lead in the ventricle, but it's something I probably **need to talk about in the future.** Right now I think it's unlikely enough, and I am not going to worry about it.

So I am primarily worried about something I can acutely change, and that would be ventilation. If I subsequently think she is losing volume in her right chest, I would initiate volume therapy, **knowing that I don't know the diagnosis.** But at this point, I need to give her volume whether she has volume loss in her right chest, a tension pneumothorax, or cardiac tamponade. **Volume will help all three.** [9]

You look at the chest x-ray and determine that the patient has a 10% pneumothorax on the left side. The cardiac silhouette is indeterminate. The pressure is now 40/palp.

The major things I am thinking about are the three I already mentioned. They are all consistent with her losing volume into her right chest. They are also consistent with pneumothorax and a cardiac tamponade.

I would continue to give her volume, intubate her, and pop a needle into her right chest. I would make sure that she has volume and see whether I can get blood out. The difficulty with putting a needle in her right chest is that I am not convinced that it's going to help her. Maybe we'll get volume out—it's going to help her. [10]

This patient needs control of her airway and volume repletion, even before I make the diagnosis. [11]

in. [5] I wonder about her volume status at this point. We can move the catheter out of the ventricle and see if that has affected her pressure. These are the two initial steps that I would think about, especially with the difficulty in getting a subclavian started.

She needs a chest tube. [3] If she is oxygenating adequately, she does not need a chest tube. She needs a chest tube because I am worried about pneumothorax.

You have to correct her pneumothorax. Go ahead and put in a chest tube. See if you get a lot of blood back.

Think about getting a pericardiocentesis. [6]

Surgical Observations

1st-Year Resident

1 The first-year resident knows not to do a subclavian stick on the opposite side without a chest x-ray to check for pneumothorax.

2 It is highly unlikely that a hematoma from subclavian vein is not obvious externally.

3 A 10% pneumothorax will not produce shock.

3rd-Year Resident

4 One cannot put any meaningful pressure on the subclavian artery externally.

5 The resident correctly "winds back the video" to the difficult and unsuccessful subclavian stick.

6 The third-year resident suddenly realizes that there is another possibility. See the discussion of insight, the "aha phenomenon," in chapter 9 of *Surgical Intuition*, the companion book to this text.

Attending Surgeon

7 Once the attending surgeon discovers that the patient is in trouble, he makes up a very short list of three possibilities: tension pneumothorax, bleeding into the right chest from the subclavian stick, or perforated right ventricle. He thinks that the third possibility is unlikely. This guides him throughout his decision-making process. Once he has that list, he is not easily swayed from it by any other information coming in.

8 The surgeon has now mentally reviewed (in order of frequency of occurrence): (1) tension pneumothorax; (2) hypovolemic bleeding into thorax; (3) catheter-induced arrhythmia; and (4) cardiac tamponade due to catheter perforation of ventricle.

9 The surgeon began thinking about therapy very early on and mentally scanned the three likely problems again. He noted aloud that fluid therapy would help all three. Thus he did not need a specific hypothesis of what the diagnosis was. He could "forward think" and go to critical points of therapy without having a hypothesis.

10 The surgeon is now beginning to make "tests" for hard data to support the specific diagnosis.

11 This scenario shows the classic "forward thinking" of an experienced surgeon—that is, he devises a therapy that will help any of the diagnostic possibilities while continuing to work on the diagnosis.

The master surgeon does not rely on rules of thumb to deal with a failed procedure.

Cognitive Psychologist's Commentary: Pacemaker Complication

Very evident in these think-alouds is the difference between the residents and the master surgeon in the complexity of the ideas they bring to bear on the problem. Although all three are oriented to the possible damage done by a needle misaimed during a subclavicular stick, the residents' conceptions of what is wrong, and hence what should be done, are much simpler than the master surgeon's.

One element of the residents' thinking is their use of rules of thumb—things to keep in mind to help you avoid trouble. The first-year resident knows to reinsert from the same side (see Surgical Observations). The third-year resident knows that when there is initial trouble in executing a procedure, one should expect that even when the procedure appears to have succeeded, something may still be wrong. In the patient with pacemaker complications, for example, there were three opportunities for something to be damaged—and in each case the effects might become apparent only later. Although a rule of thumb may provide essential guidance when one is not highly familiar with the situation, it does not substitute for full knowledge—it is just a thumb when a whole hand is needed.

Whereas the expert surgeon recognizes a number of possibilities—bleeding into left or right chest, leak from left or right lung, cardiac tamponade, puncture of heart—the residents consider a smaller number; hence the problems they pose to themselves are less complicated. Whereas the residents think of controlling bleeding by putting pressure on the chest, the expert surgeon thinks how he can discover whether covert bleeding is taking place by checking the patient's mental status and monitoring her vital signs. For example, tachycardia could confirm blood loss into the right chest, but the absence of tachycardia would not eliminate it.

When new information is received—left pneumothorax and indeterminate cardiac silhouette—the first-year resident focuses on the first piece of information only,[1] proposing a chest tube as a response to the pneumothorax. The third-year resident responds to each piece of information in turn. First, he proposes a chest tube to correct the pneumothorax, then he thinks about investigating the heart for tamponade. His thinking shows continuity with what went before, because he recognizes that the chest tube may also reveal accumulated blood. The expert surgeon's thinking shows much more continuity with his previous perception of the situation. He has the three possibilities in mind simultaneously—right chest bleeding, pneumothorax, and cardiac tamponade. Some of the ideas he considers are related to more than one possible diagnosis. For example, volume resuscitation will help, no matter which of the three is the correct diagnosis.

With the expert surgeon's ability to sketch a "big picture" for the patient and keep it in mind, he does not spend as much time as the residents in reacting to the latest finding.

---

1. Abernathy CM, Hamm RM: Surgical Intuition. Philadelphia, PA, Hanley & Belfus, 1994, chapter 4.

31. SOLITARY PULMONARY NODULE

A 72-year-old man presents with a peripheral, noncalcified 3-cm nodule in his right upper lung field. How would you manage this patient?

2nd-Year Resident

I'd do a history and physical, looking for a history of smoking, any neoplasms, and past medical history. I would look at his chest x-ray if it came with him. I would get a CT scan of the chest, looking for other smaller lesions that might not have shown up on the plain film as well as for lymph nodes. Next I would get tissue for diagnosis. Needle aspiration would not be enough—cytology is not definitive because it's not really tissue. Then I would proceed with thoracotomy and resection of the nodule. ☐

Chief Resident

I'd want to get a history and physical exam. In particular, I would want to know whether he has had a previous chest x-ray, and if so, when. The nodule may have been there before, and I want to know if it's changed. I'd want to get a history of smoking and tuberculosis or other infectious diseases. In the physical exam I'd want to know about lymph nodes. I'd want to make sure he didn't have evidence of pneumonia or other infectious process. Then the nodule: is it so peripheral that you think it's on the far chest wall?

If it's completely surrounded by a rim of lung tissue, the next step is to proceed with bronchoscopy and get the washings or biopsy—if the nodule is accessible. I would discuss with the radiologist the possibility of a biopsy with a needle through the chest wall. And I would get a CT scan. There is a chance of pneumothorax. ☐

Attending Surgeon

The first thing I would do is to take a careful history. I want to know about any exposures, any infectious agents—tuberculosis, for example—in the area the patient is from. Could the nodule possibly be due to a fungal agent in the histo belt of the Appalachian Kentucky area or the cocci belt in the Southwest. I want to know his smoking history, any industrial exposures to asbestos—that type of thing. I would ask about his **last chest x-ray** before the current one to see if this was a new or an expanded lesion. If it's been there obviously for a long period of time and hasn't changed, it is likely to be a benign lesion. If it's a new or expanding lesion, then you think of a probable malignancy.

Those would be my starting points. With a new chest lesion in anybody over the age of 40, it's **cancer until proved otherwise**. It has at least a 40 or 50% chance of being cancer, and the risk is even higher in the common smoking population.

After the history, the physical, and the review of percentages, you decide that you need to investigate the nodule to find out if it is cancer. How would you go about that?

The first time I see the patient, if I see him as an outpatient, I would ask for a collection of **2 or 3 early-morning sputums**. This is a noninvasive way that sometimes gives you an answer—positive cytology or cultures.

If the sputum specimens are negative, I need more information. I would go to bronchoscopy, probably fiberoptic **bronchoscopy**. This is a very peripheral lesion. I would do the bronchoscopy under fluoroscopic control so that I could be sure that I was brushing out in the area of the tumor. If it's a proximal lesion, I would try to identify it visually and then do the biopsy.

At the same time, or even possibly before I did the bronchoscopy, I would go ahead with a **CT scan**. There are two major reasons for the CT scan: (1) to **identify** any enlarged mediastinal **lymph nodes** and (2) to find out some **characteristics of the primary mass itself**, such as calcium density, and involvement of the chest wall. The CT should cover the chest and the upper abdomen because with one study you can get an idea—not an absolute answer by any means but an idea—not only of possible mediastinal lymphadenopathy but also of possible liver or adrenal metastases. Those are two of the three most common extrathoracic metastases—the brain is the most common. Usually in the absence of neurologic symptoms, I would not get a brain scan or CT of the brain.

If the lymph nodes are enlarged—and by enlarged radiologists usually mean greater than 1 cm—then you would have an extra suspicion of metastatic spread of a tumor through the lymph nodes. That is the way I would progress. I might want to do mediastinoscopy in the same setting. It depends to a degree on the clinical set-up—whether you're going to do the bronchoscopy on an outpatient basis. [6]

This is a peripheral lesion? You still have to assume it is cancer until proved otherwise. At this point, I would go to a fine-needle aspiration unless the lesion is located in such a spot that our radiology colleagues are afraid that the risk/benefit ratio would be too risky. I'd go to **fine-needle aspiration** at this point.

You have decided to do a thoracotomy. You open the chest and palpate the 3-cm nodule in the right upper lobe. You notice a number of enlarged mediastinal nodes. You remove one, and the pathologist returns a report of adenocarcinoma.

2nd-Year Resident

Whether or not the whole thing is resectable depends, I think—I am not familiar with this stage—on how close it is to the hilum, whether it touches the lateral side. I know they're different zones, but I am not sure which are which. ②

We are taking you rather far for the second-year level. Does the attending have any comments on what the resident did?

Attending: I wouldn't have been quite as fast to move to an operation. You make the case that everything is negative, but that you have to explore the patient because there's a chance of cancer. But I would try to go with a bronchoscopy or a needle. If the pathologist reported small-cell cancer, I wouldn't operate on the patient. I'd ask my medical oncologist to treat him with combined chemotherapy and radiation and so forth. That's one reason to confirm a diagnosis.

If the pathologist reports a specific disease entity on the basis of your fine-needle aspiration, that's fairly solid—roughly, about 80% or so certainty that the diagnosis is correct. The problem comes when the fine-needle aspiration brings back a report of non-specific cancer. Then you have to explore the patient. You may do some unnecessary thoracotomies. It depends on your philosophy. You can say, "I think I'd rather take out some granulomas than miss a cancer," but I think you could end up operating on some patients with small-cell cancer.

Chief Resident

His chest is open, and he has good pulmonary function tests. Is the nodule something I can wedge out? It is unresectable, I think, if the patient has enlarged mediastinal nodes. ④ But I already submitted him to a thoracotomy to find that out. The lesion is really peripheral, so the chance that he's going to have postoperative pneumonia is low. ⑤ I would take it out.

Any comments from the attending surgeon?

Perhaps one could make a case, in a patient who is 72 and has a 3-cm tumor, that the lesion is right on the border between T1 and T2. **Possibly you could make a case for doing a mediastinoscopy even if you had a negative CT.** Across the board, **if you skip the mediastinoscopy because you have a negative CT, you will be wrong about 16 or 17% of the time.** In other words, the nodes will be of normal size but **still have tumor.** If they are going to clean out nodes anyway, most people don't let that bother them. They say, "I can just clean them out."

Attending Surgeon

First of all, I would hope to avoid this situation by properly staging the patient before I opened the chest. I would have **done a mediastinoscopy** and perhaps found the positive nodes. Then there are several approaches to the patient. If you identify positive mediastinal node disease ahead of time, you can make the case that if the nodes are not confluent and not immobile; you can perform a lobectomy and resection of the primary tumor and a radical lymph node dissection. Then you follow the surgery with radiation and/or chemotherapy. Or you could make the case that the probability of survival is decreased to the point that you should just treat the patient with radiation or chemotherapy, or a combination of the two.

In the same area where you're already in the chest, I would go ahead with **resection of the primary tumor and clean out the lymph nodes** if at all possible. Probably I would treat the patient with adjuvant therapy postoperatively—a combination of chemotherapy and perhaps radiation therapy. One reason for trying to identify such patients up front is that our institution participates in Southwest Oncology Protocols. We try to identify subsegments of patients who may benefit from combined modality therapy. If we identify them ahead of time, we may elect to give them neoadjuvant therapy, which means preoperative chemotherapy or preoperative chemotherapy plus radiation to shrink the tumor.

Attending Surgeon *(Continued)*

If the patient has a complete or partial response—in other words, if the patient shows some sensitivity to treatment, we go ahead and operate. If I think I can clean out the nodes, I would go ahead and resect the nodes. Would I do a wedge resection☐ if it were possible? The only cancer group studying T1 and T0 lesions with wedge or segmental resection vs. lobectomy reports a higher rate of local recurrence in patients with a limited resection rather than a lobectomy. But the study is not over yet in terms of long-term follow-up; the survival statistics are not yet known.

Would it change your approach if we had made the lesion a squamous cancer as opposed to an adenocarcinoma?

Adenocarcinoma doesn't have as good a prognosis. If I knew about the mediastinal nodes preoperatively, I probably would not have operated on the patient, or I would have put the patient on a protocol with preoperative adjuvant therapy. If I am in the situation you are talking about, if I'm already in the chest, my approach wouldn't change. I'd go ahead with the resection.

Surgical Observations

2nd-Year Resident

1. The resident is doing well and wants to get to the OR but jumps ahead without knowing the exact reliability of data from a needle aspirate of a lung nodule.

2. The resident correctly tries to frame the problem with "staging" so that he might be able to relate it to something he has read. The "stage" is the bridge between the clinical findings and the literature.

Chief Resident

3. The chief resident is unaware that a pneumothorax would be an "acceptable" complication in view of the potential information the biopsy would provide.

4. The chief resident talks correctly about mediastinal nodes, but he doesn't ask the right question of himself—that is, how are we actually going to determine if the patient has enlarged mediastinal nodes? With mediastinoscopy? With CT? With mediastinoscopy only if CT shows node > 1 cm? The *answerable* questions must be asked.

   The resident also is confused about the difference between "unresectability" and "not likely to be curative."

5. The chief resident is correct to see the value of both cure and palliation.

Attending Surgeon

6. The attending surgeon exhibits the structuring of the work-up—what tests and so forth should be done—according to whether he wants to turn the work-up *against* thoracotomy (i.e., more liberal with mediastinoscopy) or for thoracotomy (which usually *requires* less work-up and shows the willingness to take more risk for a small and poorly defined chance of cure.)

Continued on following page.

7 The attending anticipates the wedge vs. lobectomy question. This question probably would be in his mind in the OR, and he would tailor the decision to the patient—i.e., poor risk vs. good risk, marginal pulmonary function, and so forth. Randomized studies would not guide him at this point in the OR; technical considerations and the like would be foremost in his mind.

It is difficult to explain one's expert judgment.

Cognitive Psychologist's Commentary: Solitary Pulmonary Nodule

In the expert surgeon's thoughts and explanations about this case we can see in action a form of intuition—judgments that the surgeon cannot fully explain. The judgments could be described, however, through psychologists' objective methods, based on observation of a number of decisions in similar situations.

Attending's explanations of his judgments. The expert surgeon explains the basis for a number of decisions in the management of the pulmonary nodule. These explanations sketch the landscape: the important features (pulmonary nodes, node locations, lymph nodes in mediastinum) and the general relations among these features (more or larger pulmonary nodes → worse prognosis; mediastinal lymph node involvement → worse prognosis). The surgeon also explains strategies that would be used in specific circumstances (how to determine the stage before operating; different techniques for sampling peripheral or proximal pulmonary lesions).

Within this broad landscape, the surgeon says that some of the decisions require individual judgment. In these situations, tradeoffs must be made between competing risks and morbidities, or the usual recommended response may not be done because of special characteristics of the patient, such as age. For example, in deciding whether to examine the patient with the mediastinoscope even if the CT shows no enlarged lymph nodes in the mediastinum, one adjusts the decision on the basis of the patient's age: "In a 72-year-old you may want to weigh that." The surgeon (in Surgical Observation 7) points out another example: the decision about wedge biopsy vs. lobectomy would be tailored to the patient on the basis of such factors as good or poor risk and quality of pulmonary function.

The surgeon's explanation of how these decisions are made is not very specific. He can identify what has to be weighed and the qualitative relation (the more of this, the more of that: e.g., the more mediastinal node involvement, the worse the prognosis), but he gives no indication of the tradeoff rate. For example, for taking a wedge versus a whole lobe, how **much** advantage (the higher probability of getting all the cancer with the lobectomy) does it take to offset the attendant disadvantage (greater morbidity due to taking a larger piece of lung)?

The actual process by which these judgments are made is covert to the expert. His naming of the important factors and constraints does not in fact describe the judgment process in a way that would allow the resident to make the same judgment if both were presented with another case.[1]

Judgments: integration of multiple inputs. To understand the surgeon's judgments, we need to review the nature of the decision problems and how people think about them. Formal analysis of these decisions[2] indicates that the best choice is a function of a number of factors that can vary continuously. Whether to open the chest for the pulmonary nodule depends simultaneously on how far the disease has progressed, on how frail the patient is, and on other factors that are not "yes or no" but rather a matter of degree. Formal models of such situations define a "decision variable," which is a continuous function of the relevant factors. If any of the factors changes a little bit, then the decision variable changes a little bit. Then decisions can be made by defining points or thresholds for the decision variable: "if it is above point T, operate." In such situations, the factors sometimes compete and have to be traded off against each other. While factor A might be high enough to push the average patient beyond the threshold of operating, factors B and C may be below average. Thus the decision variable is still below the threshold.

Experts do not have such statistical models in their heads, but they act as if they do[3]; that is, the judgments that they make about patients can be described with models of this sort. In one study,[4] physicians with different levels of experience (third-year medical students, first- and third-year residents, and active clinicians with at least 5 years clinical experience) were asked to make judgments about 27 hypothetical patients: Does the patient have pulmonary embolus? Would you initiate anticoagulation therapy? The patient descriptions were constructed of 8 factors related to pulmonary embolus that could vary among cases, including heart rate, respiration rate, PO_2 and extent of defects on perfusion scan. The levels of the factors were systematically varied across the 27 case descriptions so that the influence of each factor on the physician's judgment could be determined.

Statistical analysis of each physician's judgments—using the 8 factors to predict the judgment whether the patient had a pulmonary embolus—produced a model with a number of significant features. First, the model described how the physician combined the various factors into an overall judgment as a "weighted average." Second, the weights from the model serve as an approximate measure of the importance of each factor in the physician's judgments. Third, the weights can be used to describe tradeoffs between the different factors—for example, in the physician's judgment of whether patients have pulmonary embolus, an increase of one unit on one factor may be offset by a decrease of two units on another factor. Finally, the models can differ from each other with respect to the relative weights the physicians put on the factors and hence the tradeoffs they make between factors.

Usually people who make these sorts of judgments have no idea how they do it. Without an analysis such as that used in the pulmonary embolus study, there would be no way to determine the weights or tradeoffs. Sometimes people use the vocabulary of such analysis in a qualitative manner: "I put more weight on the lung scan than the PO_2 when I make that judgment." But this is almost like comparing two runners who ran different courses without measuring the distances or elapsed times.

A number of studies have focused on people's judgments of various concepts. Usually simple mathematical models—weighted averages of the features—are sufficient to describe the judgments, particularly when the participants' explanations of the situation focus only on which features are important.[5] If their explanations include branching sequences of decisions—rules prescribing that different things be done in different situations—then more complex models may be required to describe the resulting judgments.[6]

In light of such results, it is not surprising that the expert surgeon in this case cannot give a more precise description of the judgments he makes, beyond what factors are important. To be more specific, he would need to use a precise technical vocabulary[1,2] to specify the relations in a way that could be communicated and reproduced. Most expert surgeons probably do not know that vocabulary, and surely they do not think in such terms when making their judgments—they are aware of the judgments, not of the process. Moreover, the residents would not be able to interpret advice stated in such a vocabulary.

Learning expert judgment. How, then, do residents learn to make expert judgments? Learning takes place when they think about particular cases and about how to handle the disease in general. With particular patients, residents learn from experience—what happens in their own and others' cases—and from watching how experts think about such cases (including reading this sort of think-aloud).

Considering the problem at the general level provides another avenue for learning expert judgment. Residents can learn from several sorts of information. First, they can be told in general what factors are important in a situation—what should get more weight in a tradeoff. Recalling this information can guide them when they actually have to make the tradeoffs. Second, they could learn to use numerical indices. For example, Gregory et al.[7] present a system for grading the severity of mangled extremities. The system involves assigning a score to each of 8 dimensions, then adding them up: if total is more than 20, then amputate. This index has the same form as the statistical models that describe people's judgments; implicit in the index is the kind of tradeoff discussed above. The surgeon who has mastered the use of such a formula may not be able to discuss tradeoffs formally—to specify numerically how much of a difference in one dimension (e.g., nerve function) compensates for how much of a difference in bone damage. But because this tradeoff is implicit in the formula, when the resident has internalized the scale, then his or her judgments implicitly handle the tradeoff between the dimensions.

Another method for teaching expert judgment involves cognitive feedback.[8] The residents are shown the weights in the model that describe how they currently make the judgments, and these weights are compared with those that describe the expert's judgments. Thus the residents can know to which factors they are paying too much or too little attention.

Systematic probing of memory. The chief resident "drew a blank" when given the second description of this case. Faced with the dilemma, he waited for the script concerning what to do in this situation to come to mind. When no pattern came immediately, he managed his long-term working memory to direct the mental search thoroughly, within the limitations of working memory capacity.[9] By repeating key phrases that described the situation, he refreshed the information in his short-term memory, where it could serve as a probe to stimulate the search of his long-term memory. By repeating aspects of the situation that he had not mentioned recently, he put in mind novel combinations of information about the patient that may have triggered different patterns. Although he finished by feeling rather lame, he had done the right thing: he stopped and allowed his mind the time to do the searching necessary to find the pattern if it had been there.

1. Abernathy CM, Hamm RM: Surgical Intuition. Philadelphia, PA, Hanley & Belfus, 1994, chapter 8.
2. Abernathy CM, Hamm RM: Surgical Intuition. Philadelphia, PA, Hanley & Belfus, 1994, chapter 7.
3. Hoffman PJ: The paramorphic representation of clinical judgment. Psychol Bull 57:116–131, 1960.
4. Wigton RS, Hoellerich VL, Patil KD: How physicians use clinical information in diagnosing pulmonary embolism: An application of conjoint analysis. Med Decision Making 6:2–11, 1986.
5. Dawes RM: The robust beauty of improper linear models. Am Psychol 34:571–582, 1979.
6. Hamm RM: Modeling expert forecasting knowledge for incorporation in expert systems. J Forecasting 12:117–137, 1993.
7. Gregory RT, Gould RJ, Peclet M, et al: The mangled extremity syndrome (M.E.S.): A severity grading system for multisystem injury of the extremity. J Trauma 25:1147–1150, 1985.
8. Hammond KR, Summers DA, Deane DH: Negative effects of outcome-feedback in multiple-cue probability learning. Organizat Behav Hum Perform 9:30–34, 1973.
9. Abernathy CM, Hamm RM: Surgical Intuition. Philadelphia, PA, Hanley & Belfus, 1994, chapter 4.

32. SEPSIS OF UNKNOWN FOCUS

In the intensive care unit you see a 57-year-old woman who underwent gastric resection 10 days ago. She has a fever spiking to 39° C daily; her white blood cell count is 12,500; her chest x-ray shows bilateral infiltrates; her sputum has multiple organisms with many white cells; and she is on the ventilator. The CT scan of her abdomen is nondiagnostic. What are your thoughts about this patient?

1st-Year Resident

I would assess neurologic status and then would move on to other systems. She is on the ventilator? I would look at her **oxygenation and ventilation;** obviously of concern are her pulmonary infiltrates. I don't know if they are lobar or panlobar infiltrates diffusely on both sides. The picture is consistent with **ARDS**—the fever, white cell count and sputum. I also would be worried about some type of **hospital-acquired pneumonia,** and I would want to review cultures to see how legitimate her sputum sample may be in regard to white cells. I would worry about sepsis, and I would want to know some of her **hemodynamic values** to see if she fits in that category. If she didn't have a Swan-Ganz catheter, I would recommend inserting one to get some numbers and to follow her pulmonary wedge pressure and systemic vascular resistance. From a GI standpoint, if she's postoperative day 10, she could have a breakdown of her anastomosis or some type of wound infection.

3rd-Year Resident

My initial concern would be that she could have an **anastomotic dehiscence** [1] from her gastric hook-up. For example, if she had a Billroth II anastomosis, she may have a **duodenal stump blow-out.** [2] I wouldn't necessarily ascribe the findings to atelectasis. [3] I might pursue a Gastrografin study to rule out extravasation. The positive findings on her chest x-ray were bilateral infiltrates, she is a little tachycardic, and she has a white cell count of 12,000. Certainly extravasation could account for the findings, but I would not make that assumption. My next step would be a Gastrografin study and evaluation of the anastomosis.

Attending Surgeon

I would want to know her **clinical course** [4]—whether there has been a sudden deterioration, one, from a sepsis standpoint and, two, from a pulmonary standpoint. [5] The big question going through my mind is, **"Does she have pneumonia, or does she have an intraabdominal disaster?"** The latter would probably represent a leak, and the CT scan, although helpful, doesn't necessarily rule it out. [6] I would aim my diagnostic work-up toward understanding what her response and her course have been and how she is responding to whatever therapy has been instituted. I would imagine that they are concerned that she has pneumonia and have started her on antibiotics.

I would be concerned about her wound. If she had an open wound, I would take cultures. I also would take blood cultures.

You've seen the patient and written your consulting report. She has been on multiple antibiotics, and 4 more days have passed. Now she has gone from alert to comatose, her bilirubin has increased from normal to 8, she remains febrile, and her white blood cell count remains 12,500.

Neurologically, she has gone from awake to comatose. Now her bilirubin is up, she's still febrile, and her white cell count is still up. Something may have been missed initially that would be consistent with multiorgan failure at this point. Her comatose state could be due to a **ventilation-oxygenation problem, low perfusion,** or liver failure, all of which are consistent with sepsis—if we're going to think about sepsis. I would want to look at a lot of her numbers from a pulmonary artery catheter to make that diagnosis. I would question her antibiotics. If her antibiotics are still the same and we're not getting much response, it may be something else, such as a systemic fungus infection.

She's obviously septic from some focus, and that accounts for her change in mental status and most likely for her elevated bilirubin—isolated elevation of bilirubin in a patient that is obviously very septic. Probably the **only focus of sepsis that could account for that degree of change is either in her abdomen or in her chest**—but her chest x-ray has not worsened. With that limited information, 4 days later, I think you have two options: (1) to explore her abdomen and rule out a septic focus in the abdomen or (2) to restudy her in some other way, such as repeat CT of the abdomen. If she's stable enough to take down to the scanner, that's a reasonable option.

That would be rather alarming, because I would expect that most bacterial pneumonia—if they selected the appropriate broad-spectrum antibiotics and have gotten back culture-dated results—should be resolving. **She wouldn't be going into multiple organ failure (MOF) from that.** Abnormal bile stasis goes with sepsis, as do MOF and liver function, but I would be very concerned that I was putting too much credence in the fact that she had pneumonia. Would I rush her to the operating room? That's a tough question because she probably will not tolerate a negative exploration. Therefore I may choose to do some sort of **Gastrografin swallow,** something that demonstrates a leak. Again, **a lot of decisions depend on what her course has been.** But you're describing multiple organ failure, and **things aren't going to get better unless something changes.**

Surgical Observations

3rd-Year Resident

[1] The third-year resident brings up the "surgically correctable" leaking anasto-mosis earlier in his thinking than the first-year resident, who focuses on general sepsis management.

[2] The third-year resident has more "domain-specific" knowledge. He reviews in his mind what the operation might have been. A master surgeon would go even further and review *every detail* (e.g., sutures, size of bites, "angle of death") of the operation in his or her mind (replay the video).

[3] The third-year resident remembers not to use a "waste-basket" diagnosis, such as atelectasis or aspiration, which may prevent him from finding the true cause of sepsis.

Attending Surgeon

[4] The attending invokes the *timing* and temporal relationships of the patient's course; that is, he does not look just at the present slice of time.

[5] The attending has clearly pitted abdominal vs. pulmonary sepsis as the two diagnoses he must distinguish between.

[6] The attending realizes the limitations of the data.

The expert builds a mental model of the patient's system.

Cognitive Psychologist's Commentary: Sepsis of Unknown Focus

In the least pleasant of all dilemmas, any option is bad. The physician has a patient in serious trouble that could be due to pneumonia, sepsis from the gastric resection area, or both. She may need an operation, yet she may not be able to tolerate it.

The first-year resident's recognition of the patterns in this case is a slow and unsteady process, and he or she resorts to repetition of the information to help fix it in mind long enough to trigger the matching categories from memory: "Neurologically, she has gone from awake to comatose. Now her bilirubin is up, she's still febrile, and her white cell count is still up." Whereas the more experienced physicians can process these details as they are read, the first-year resident needs to rehearse them to ensure that they will stay in mind long enough for their meaning to be appreciated and for them to serve as stimuli for pattern recognition to retrieve other ideas from long-term memory.[1] The resident is developing a system for storing the information in extended long-term memory, as if on different labeled shelves: "Neurologically, she has gone from awake to comatose." This mental structure for sorting and storing the facts of the case supports more reliable retrieval of information.[2]

The surgeons at all three levels of experience recognize the diagnostic dilemma—abdominal sepsis vs. pulmonary sepsis. The first-year resident mentions possibilities and procedures that the others would not even consider, Swan-Ganz catheter and neurologic exam. He has not yet mastered the conventional scripts, in particular the ability to judge relative importance within the scripts.

Only the expert surgeon focuses on *control:* "I would aim my diagnostic work-up toward understanding what her response and her course have been and how she is responding to whatever therapy has been initiated." These responses will help the expert to figure out the source of the sepsis. But they also give a sense of where the patient is and how responsive she will be to any interventions. The expert is not simply remembering facts about the patient, filed in a set of labeled shelves. He is building a model of the patient that represents how she has responded to resuscitations and interventions so far and also how she would respond to other interventions.

The expert surgeon's model covers what has happened, what is happening now, and what may happen next. The surgeon needs to see how much of his various external inputs (e.g., fluid, antibiotics) have been required to maintain her present condition. He has in mind a spectrum or ladder for each of these external inputs. For example, at the bottom of the antibiotics ladder are the single-agent, narrow-spectrum drugs and at the top are the broad-spectrum drugs, the big guns kept in reserve.

When managing a patient or interpreting a patient's course, the surgeon thinks in terms of setting the fluids at the right amount—not too much (overload will add to sepsis problems) and not too little (the opportunity for improving her status will be missed). He finds an optimal point. The position of the current optimal point on the ladder of antibiotics, for example, is an important indicator not only of the seriousness of the patient's condition but also of what kind of control is available if needed. The more extreme the position on each input, the less flexibility he has for control. And when the patient is very inflexible on one input, there is probably not much resiliency on the others.

Reasoning about systems requires a special kind of mental model. How much of a change in one input (e.g., fluids) is required to produce a given amount of change in another output (e.g., cardiac output)? Which inputs or combinations of inputs can be used to control a particular output, and which are completely ineffective?

The ability to use such models is a mark of expertise.[3] They transcend categorical responses and provide a flexible understanding of the situation that can be used to respond to or to anticipate any change.[4] And in the present dilemma, the model provides the expert surgeon with a basis for a decision uniquely appropriate for this patient. The categorical recognitions of the residents are not as useful.

---

1. Abernathy CM, Hamm RM: Surgical Intuition. Philadelphia, PA, Hanley & Belfus, 1994, chapters 3 and 4.
2. Ericsson KA, Kintsch W: Memory in comprehension and problem solving: A long-term working memory. Boulder, CO, Institute of Cognitive Science, University of Colorado Press, 1991.
3. Abernathy CM, Hamm RM: Surgical Intuition. Philadelphia, PA, Hanley & Belfus, 1994, chapter 8.

33. LIVER LACERATION FROM MOTOR VEHICLE ACCIDENT

A 69-year-old woman is brought to the emergency department after a motor vehicle accident. She was wearing restraints. Her BP is 90/60, pulse is 120 bpm. Radiographs of the cervical spine, pelvis, and chest are negative. DPL shows 50,000 red blood cells per cc, and the urine is blood-tinged. How would you manage this case?

3rd-Year Resident

First, I would begin with the ABCs. I'd make sure that the patient had adequate airways and no neurologic disability. I'd use universal precautions and make sure that the patient's breathing and ventilation are adequate and that she has an adequate level of consciousness. Then I would assess circulation and begin my initial resuscitation. Because the patient is hypotensive and tachycardic, I am concerned that a significant amount of blood has been lost from somewhere. **It sounds like the DPL is not fully explained,** □ so I would begin two large-bore peripheral IV's for fluid resuscitation. Then I'd go back for my secondary survey and try to identify any other potential areas of blood loss.

Chief Resident

The patient shows signs of blood loss, hypotension and tachycardia. She is also elderly, and you have to worry about cardiac contusion because you haven't told me **where they are hiding that amount of blood.** The chest x-ray is clear, so it's unlikely that you could account for any significant blood loss above the diaphragm. Peritoneal lavage suggests that there isn't a large amount of blood in the abdomen, □ and the blood-tinged urine suggests a retroperitoneal process. She may have renal injury. Again, to lose the amount of blood necessary to cause class 3 shock makes me concerned about the abdomen, the peritoneal cavity. I would begin actively resuscitating the patient and probably get a one-shot IVP in the ED, with the concern that she may have a renal vascular injury. If that were normal, I would be able to stabilize the patient. I would probably proceed with a cystogram.

Attending Surgeon

The very first consideration is the vital signs. Because the systolic pressure of 90 with a heart rate of 120 tends to imply hypovolemia, I would be vigilant for a source of ongoing blood loss when she arrives. The chest x-ray, the DPL, and the pelvic x-ray would be the types of things I would look for to corroborate the concern for hypovolemia. □ After finding the source of blood loss, I would move to my second concern—**the source of relative hypotension** and relative tachycardia. I would ascertain the validity of this concern by looking at her response to fluids. With a red-cell contamination of 50,000 on DPL—and I presume this is a good DPL—the **next thing I would do is challenge the data** because they're not making sense. □ I would like to know (1) **how she responds to fluid,** (2) her **hematocrit,** and (3) her relative cardiac pulmonary function. Is she on medications, or does she have evidence of myocardial contusion?

You order a second DPL, and the blood pressure has dropped to the 60 level. You decide to go to the OR. You have done a midline laparotomy, you've mopped out 1,000 cc of blood, and you notice that the only intraoperative finding is a 3-inch-deep laceration of the dome of the right lobe of the liver. The patient has received 6 units of blood. The laceration is actively bleeding.

At this point, I would start by **finger-fracturing the laceration** further, identifying the bleeding points, and attempting to oversew the larger bleeding points. ②

And if it's still actively bleeding?

At that point, I would perform a Pringle maneuver to get temporary control of the bleeding and try to oversew the bleeding points.

At this point, you want to mobilize the liver by taping down the triangular ligament and **try to apply pressure to control the bleeding so that you can resuscitate the patient.** ②

Then you're faced with more definitive control. I would probably start some finger-fracturing to see if I can get in there and suture-ligate the bleeders. I would consider performing a Pringle maneuver if I couldn't get enough control to see what is bleeding. The other alternative would be a Longmire clamp to control the bleeding, then suture ligation of the vessels. But if this procedure is extended deep enough, you'd be down in the hepatic veins, and you'd have to try another plan.

Tell me about her vital signs again and her response to fluid.

She's had 6 units of blood. Her blood pressure is 60, her heart rate 160.

Again, you face the issue of synthesizing the data and their sources. If the BP is 60 and the heart rate 160, the immediate concern is to find out what can be transpiring that is remedial. **I wouldn't get distracted by the fracture in the right lobe of the liver.** ② The thought of a caval injury would enter my mind. First of all, I would put tubes in both sides of the chest and do a pericardial window before I'd worry about the liver.

The pericardial window is negative, and the chest tubes have minimal blood coming out of them, but by now the laceration in the liver is pouring blood.

That suggests a diagnosis of caval injury, although the initial presentation of 1,000 cc of blood in the abdomen would challenge that diagnosis, ④ suggesting that it may be compounded by air embolism. But the fact is, you now have a sufficient known blood loss in the peritoneal cavity to explain the hemodynamics, and I would prepare for retroperitoneal injury.

How would you do that?

The first thing would be to **summon help.** ⑤ My first priority is to get a second-year resident to help me and an attending anesthesiologist to resuscitate the patient. The second thing is to look around the table and see who is there to help. If I'm with a second- or third- year resident and doing a stab wound to the liver as well, I want the nurses to start calling for help. As we're

Attending Surgeon *(Continued)*

talking, **we'll pack off the liver** to stem the bleeding because if this is a retroperitoneal caval injury, the **last thing we need to do is to enter the liver too soon.** Tamponade should control the bleeding. The summons for help and packing the liver are simultaneous—they are the main priority.

The number 2 priority is resuscitation, which again depends on the constellation of the people around the table and their sophistication in anticipating what you need. If the chief resident is standing next to me, I just need to say, "We have a caval injury," and the next thing, we're done. If I am with an anesthesiologist in whom I have less than great trust, I have to start balancing what I am going to do to the liver against educating the anesthesiologist about what we do for resuscitation. A great deal of decision making is affected by who you have around the room and how you balance that with your major priorities. The number 1 priority is resuscitation; the number 2 priority is to control the bleeding. If we have the right people, if the communication is assured, and if resuscitation is under way, the next issue is what to do with the liver. After the packs are placed around the liver, does the laceration continue to bleed? Or does the bleeding stop?

It continues to bleed.

If the bleeding continues, then **Pringle maneuver** should be performed to stem ongoing active hemorrhage from the liver and to facilitate resuscitation.

The Pringle maneuver is done, and the laceration is still bleeding.

Well, **that supports the diagnosis of retroperitoneal caval injury,**[6] if in fact the blood emanating from the liver is desaturated. That's an important issue, because you may have a hepatic artery that is not isolated with the major vessel. If you have desaturated blood after the Pringle maneuver, then you're dealing with a caval injury.[7]

Surgical Observations

3rd-Year Resident, Chief Resident, and Attending Surgeon

[1] The third-year resident is *slightly* troubled because the DPL is not "fully explained"; in other words, he's not certain what is bleeding in the abdomen. At the same point, the chief resident correlates the vital signs and the DPL and realizes that the DPL has not explained the decrease in the vital signs; nor has the chest x-ray, which he reviews in his mind. Finally, at the exact same point the attending surgeon focuses *very strongly* on the fact that the DPL definitely does not explain the vital signs, which are consistent with shock. Almost simultaneously he brings in three or four factors, such as response to fluids. He is willing to "challenge the data" (because they do not make sense) and questions the reliability of the DPL. Did enough fluid come back? Did the patient have adhesions from previous surgery that could sequester blood loss? The surgeon moves immediately to the steps he would take because the vital signs show a blood loss that is not explained. He plans to check the patient's response to fluid, her hematocrit, and her pulmonary and cardiac function, and to review the history for medications that may play a role. It bothers him greatly that two pieces of strong data are in conflict.

Continued on following page.

2 The third-year resident begins finger-fracturing the liver, focusing on the technical aspects of how he can control the bleeding. The chief resident also thinks about finger-fracturing, but first he considers techniques to mobilize the liver and application of pressure to control the bleeding so that the patient can be resuscitated. At this point the attending surgeon does not give even a fleeting thought to controlling the relatively minor liver laceration and will not let it "distract him" from trying to explain why the patient's vital signs indicate deep shock when minimal blood (1,000 cc) is seen within the peritoneal cavity. His mind scans to other areas that could be more occult, such as caval injuries. He even puts tubes in each side of the chest and does a pericardial window, stating specifically that he would take these steps before he would worry about the liver.

Attending Surgeon

3 In general, expert surgeons share three strategies in their approach to the problem of the think-aloud: (1) they concentrate intently when the problem is presented; (2) almost invariably they pause for a few seconds to absorb the information and sift it around in their heads, thinking before they begin to talk; and (3) when they begin, they have a few general thoughts about *the particular pattern* of the problem, its particular scenario, what they think the questions about this patient and the pivotal decision points are going to be.

4 The attending surgeon arrives at a possible diagnosis of air embolus, although he is beginning to accept that the problem may be a caval injury. Even though he still is not absolutely convinced, he begins to plan for repair of injury to a major vessel of the retroperitoneum.

5 The attending's scenario focused on managing a retrohepatic caval injury. Of interest, the first thing he thinks about is the big picture: he asks about his resources for anesthesia and for resuscitating the patient if even more blood is lost. His first statement about managing the lesion is "summon help."

6 Once the Pringle maneuver is done and the liver laceration is still bleeding, the attending surgeon realizes that he now has confirmatory evidence of a retroperitoneal caval injury. He has not forgotten that the original diagnosis of retroperitoneal caval injury may be wrong, and even in the heat of battle, he is chalking up yes or no evidence.

7 The attending refused to believe that the low blood pressure matched the blood loss or the negative DPL with the normal chest and pelvis films. In his thoughts he reviewed the chest and pelvis films because he didn't like the fact that the findings failed to explain the drop in vital signs. When the discovery of 1,000 cc of blood in the belly and a bleeding liver laceration didn't explain the vital signs to him, he immediately ignored the liver laceration thought-wise and rethought why the vital signs were not explained by the findings. He would not let go of that problem during his thought process. He even went so far as to put in chest tubes and do a pericardial window because he was not fooled simply by some blood in the belly. He was looking for evidence to fit the pattern of what he knew was enough blood to explain the drop in vital signs.

Metacognition tells the expert when to search for a better understanding.

Cognitive Psychologist's Commentary:
Liver Laceration from a Motor Vehicle Accident

The contrast between the expert and novice surgeons in this case shows two facets of expert thinking: knowing when you don't know what is going on and using your judgment to ask the right questions and to plan on the fly.

The ability to detect when the situation is not well understood. All three surgeons knew that they had not yet accounted for the patient's hypovolemia, but they responded differently when the laparotomy revealed the bleeding liver. The residents went into their "control-a-bleeding-liver" script, whereas the expert trauma surgeon viewed the bleeding liver as a distraction and instead focused on finding some other injury that would account for the amount of blood loss necessary to produce the patient's poor vital signs.

Residents are still acquiring their scripts. They do not have a strong sense of when a script that they recognize does not quite fit. "I don't understand it" is a common feeling for them. When they have this feeling, they don't immediately distrust the data because they always have an alternate explanation: "Maybe it is just a deficiency in my knowledge." In contrast, the expert surgeon knows the patterns well enough to recognize that when something does not quite fit, serious attention needs to be paid to the situation until the anomaly is resolved. The feeling of discomfort now plays a key role in orienting the expert to what is important in the case.[1,2]

People often sense that a written text does not make sense (see box below). The first three sentences in the story "The Marriage of Kakra" are easy to understand. The reader makes automatic inferences, such as finding the referent for "warriors" in sentence two.

The Marriage of Kakra

The Swazi tribe was at war with a neighboring tribe because of a dispute over some cattle. Among the warriors were two unmarried men named Kakra and his younger brother Gum. Kakra was killed in battle. According to tribal custom, Kakra was married subsequently to the woman Ami (Kintsch, 1979).[3]

But the fourth sentence is anomalous and cannot be handled automatically by an adult reader. (A kindergartner might listen to the story contentedly, imagining battles and weddings but not catching the anomaly.) As Resnick[4] observes:

> To know that the final sentence is anomalous, the reader must bring topical knowledge and rules of inference to bear. The reader knows, for example, that someone killed in battle is no longer alive. In addition, he or she is likely to assume that marriage requires a living

bridegroom. This leads to the inference that it is impossible for Kakra to be married after the battle. Topical knowledge and rules of inference thus lead to the sense that the passage is incomprehensible. Yet topical knowledge can also provide the basis for resolving the comprehension problem. The knowledge needed relates to ghost marriage, a tribal custom in which, when the oldest son of a family dies without heirs, his spirit is nevertheless married as planned, and his younger brother takes his place in the marriage bed until an heir is produced.

The residents in this case are like the kindergartner listening to the story: they did not notice the anomaly; they did not know that liver laceration could not account for the blood loss. The expert surgeon is like the adult reader: he recognized the anomaly. Furthermore, because he was offered the opportunity to ask for more information, he was able to focus on a likely retroperitoneal caval injury, much like the adult reader with topical knowledge of ghost marriage.

The expert's questions and plans are guided by judgments of relative importance. When first acquiring scripts, residents use them through pattern recognition: they identify the type of situation, recall the script for that situation, and do what it says they should do. Thus the residents recognized liver laceration as the identified cause of the patient's bleeding and proceeded to read from their scripts how they would manage it.

With experience surgeons become familiar with the decision points in their scripts and gain the ability to integrate all aspects of the situation by using their judgment. This is evident in two tasks the expert surgeon posed for himself. Initially, he thought of the questions that he would ask when he saw the patient. *First*, Will the pelvic x-ray and DPL reveal a source of blood loss? *Second*, Will her response to fluids be consistent with my explanation of her tachycardia and hypotension? His ranking indicates the relative importance of the questions.

Later he thought of the steps he would need to take in preparation for retroperitoneal injury. The *first* priority is to pack the liver and to summon help simultaneously, with the type of help depending on his assessment of the skills of the team already available. The *second* priority is resuscitation.

In neither judgment task does the expert merely recognize a pattern and perform an automatic response. He recognizes multiple possibilities, and as he describes it, his response will be a function of several factors that may vary, including the patient's responses to fluids, and the number and quality of assistants in the operating room.[1] The novices do not have enough experience to make such judgments, nor is their use of their knowledge automatic enough that they can simultaneously identify the situation and the usual response and adjust their response to the actual conditions.

---

1. Abernathy CM, Hamm RM: Surgical Intuition. Philadelphia, PA, Hanley & Belfus, 1994, chapter 8.
2. Abernathy CM, Hamm RM: Surgical Intuition. Philadelphia, PA, Hanley & Belfus, 1994, chapter 9.
3. Kintsch W: On modeling comprehension. Educ Psychol 14:3–14, 1979.
4. Resnick LB: Education and Learning to Think. Washington, DC, National Academy Press, 1987, pp 9–10.

34. HEMORRHAGIC PANCREATITIS

A 37-year-old alcoholic man is admitted with severe epigastric pain and an amylase of 800. His white blood cell count is 16,000; his temperature is 40° C, and his bilirubin is 8. How would you approach this patient?

Chief Resident

Initially I need as much history and as thorough a physical exam as I can get. I would order an ultrasound. Bilirubin of 8 is in the worry zone for cancer as a cause of duct obstruction— fairly high to be explained by swelling and duct constriction from pancreatitis. If you are considering pancreatitis, a white cell count of 16,000 puts him on the border for sepsis. **What's his blood sugar?**

His blood sugar is 60.

Attending Surgeon

First of all, a bilirubin of 8 and a temperature of 40 are highly suspicious for **a cholangitic picture,** whether from stone disease, alcoholic pancreatitis, gallstone pancreatitis, or a combination of the above. You have to assume that he has a stricture involving the common bile duct. He needs a **quick ultrasound** just to make sure he doesn't have dilated intra- and extrahepatic ducts, which could be consistent with chronic stricture, and to make sure he doesn't have stone disease. If he has no evidence of stone disease or ductal obstruction, you probably have to **assume that the elevated bilirubin is a manifestation of severe sepsis, which would be rather unusual in pancreatitis.** [1]

The ultrasound shows multiple gallstones. Twelve hours later the patient is frankly septic, with a severely tender upper abdominal exam. You take him to the OR to explore. At the time of exploration you find a pancreas that is diffusely enlarged by threefold, with areas of hemorrhage and necrosis.

If he has hemorrhagic necrosis, I would debride those areas and drain him widely with dependent drains.

First of all, you have to assume that he has an obstruction of the common bile duct and frank cholangitis. Depending on how sick and moribund he is, probably the safest and easiest option (although you can do a cholangiogram) is drainage of the common bile duct on the assumption that he has distal obstruction. [2] At the same time, if he truly has hemorrhagic and liquefying pancreas, I would scoop out what is there. That may or may not improve his overall status. But if the pancreas is clearly soft, necrotic, and hemorrhagic, I would scoop out what is there and put in multiple drains. He needs wide-spectrum antibiotics.

Surgical Observations

Attending Surgeon

[1] The attending gives a great deal of thought to what may be causing this particular picture, including whether or not there is ductal obstruction as well as other possibilities. She considers severe sepsis as a cause of the elevation of the bilirubin, but doubts that the sepsis is caused by pancreatitis.

[2] The surgeon scans widely, trying to think of what may be causing the problem. Although she comes up with a list of more likely and less likely hypotheses, she is unwilling to put much confidence in one or the other. Forward thinking is evident when the surgeon decides that the patient needs drainage of the common bile duct, even though she is unable to define whether or not the patient has bile duct obstruction at the time of the decision. The surgeon focuses initially on the "scoop out" of the liquefied pancreas, but spends some time thinking about the possible etiologies (whether provable or unprovable) of the patient's pancreatitis.

Explanation helps an observer learn the script.

Cognitive Psychologist's Commentary:
Hemorrhagic Pancreatitis

In this think-aloud the chief resident and the attending surgeon work with the same basic surgical script. But the attending offers more detail and explanation, which reflect her teaching role as well as her mastery of the material.

It is natural that the attending, who knows more about the possibilities in the situation, would have more to say. But her teaching role also demands that she explain her thinking in more detail. Students can learn clinical scripts quite effectively when explanation is provided,[1] and the master surgeon's explorations of the possible alternatives is a way of providing explanation.[2] Merely watching a surgeon follow the script without explanation, as the chief resident did here, is less helpful for the beginning resident.

Beyond its teaching value, the explicit exploration may lead to better patient care, if not in this particular patient then in the long run. Certainly the attending surgeon has more knowledge, as reflected in her more elaborate thinking. But thinking itself, the process of scanning possibilities, comparing, rejecting, spending time thinking about a patient, also has benefit. This is the way that knowledge comes into play, how it makes its contribution. Spending more time in informal, highly focused, rapid thinking makes the surgeon more likely to produce (1) discoveries of explanations for the patient's symptoms and (2) actions that take all possibilities into account.

1. Ahn W, Brewer WF, Mooney RJ: Schema acquisition from a single example. J Exper Psychol: Learn, Mem, Cogn 18:391–412, 1992.
2. Abernathy CM, Hamm RM: Surgical Intuition. Philadelphia, PA, Hanley & Belfus, 1994, chapter 11.

35. LAPAROSCOPIC CHOLECYSTECTOMY

A 42-year-old woman undergoes a laparoscopic cholecystectomy for symptoms of chronic cholecystitis. She has never had jaundice. When you cut the cystic duct, it seems big to you—approximately a 4-mm lumen. What are your thoughts about this finding? Would you do anything?

3rd-Year Resident

Thoughts about an enlarged cystic duct—it could be dilated for several reasons. Maybe she has some kind of obstruction in her common bile duct that is being transmitted to a large cystic duct. Or it could be her normal anatomy. I would like to know preoperatively if she has had any other studies. For example, did she have any study that visualizes her common bile duct, her hepatic duct, or her cystic duct? She has never been jaundiced, and clinically she never had a stone in the common bile duct, but I would like to know if any imaging studies showed whether she did or not.

What would you do in the OR?

In the OR, I would shoot a cystic duct cholangiogram.

And how would you do that?

I would try to do it laparoscopically.

Chief Resident

A 4-mm lumen is big. You wonder if the duct is dilated because she just passed a stone, which may explain why she does not appear jaundiced when she presents to you. ☐ I think that you need a **cholangiogram.**

How do you do that?

With a ureteral catheter. You can use a large-bore needle puncture and thread it through, just off the anterior axillary line above the umbilicus, or you can thread it through one of the ports. You want to put a clip on the distal part of the cystic duct for a small amount of traction. You make a small nick in the duct with your scissors, thread the ureteral catheter through the valves of Heister, and do the gram.

Attending Surgeon

I would make sure that I had **liver function tests** before surgery and an **ultrasound** that showed a common bile duct of normal size. **If the tests and the common bile duct were normal, I would not worry about a 4-mm cystic duct.** ☐

The cystic duct cholangiogram shows a normal biliary tree except for a radiolucent defect that is 4 mm in diameter, 2 cm proximal to the ampulla of Vater. What would you do?

I would see if it looks like a stone. **If it's a common bile duct stone, it needs to be dealt with in some fashion.** I could pass a basket all the way down into the duodenum, then pull it back and try to basket the stone and pull it out. That is probably what I would try to do at this point.

You want to rule out an air bubble. You can put the patient in the Trendelenberg position and shoot another cholangiogram to see if it goes away. If you're convinced that it's a stone and not an air bubble, you have two immediate options: a postoperative ERCP to try to remove the stone or a laparoscopic exploration of the common duct. Your final option, of course, is to open the patient for a common duct exploration.

And which would you do?

I would base my decision on my own and my hospital's capabilities. Personally, I would choose the ERCP because my team does it very well.

I would finish the laparoscopic cholecystectomy. A 4-mm stone might pass, but it is marginal. I would **handle the problem postoperatively with ERCP.** Ninety percent of the stones pass, and 90% of those that don't can be handled by ERCP, so only 1% of the situations you don't handle will come back to you.

A question for the attending surgeon. How would you do an operative cholangiogram during a laparoscopic cholecystectomy?

You are going to have a lot of trouble if you have already cut the duct. You said, "When you cut the cystic duct, it seems big." Hopefully you will notice that the lumen is 4 mm before you cut the duct entirely. I use the Reddick catheter. I have tried a dozen catheters, and it is by far the easiest. It has a little balloon tip. You can put it in right through the 5-mm sheath. You come in through the same hole, and you keep traction upward on the gallbladder as well as on the pouch. After you come through, you make a small nick with the scissors. The Reddick catheter has a little plastic sleeve through which goes a tiny catheter, like a little Fogarty catheter with a balloon on it. The catheter serves as a guide and goes right through the 5-mm port. You slide it in, but you don't have to get it all the way down—only far enough to blow up the balloon, which then holds itself in place. You don't have to use clamps, or clips, and the catheter has a 3-way stopcock that makes injection easy.

How do you judge how much the balloon is expanded?

You judge by direct visualization. I watch the cystic duct expand as the balloon blows up. You can overextend the balloon and rupture the duct, which gives you a real problem. I just watch until the balloon blows up and feels like it's snug (you can pull on it). It's important to insert the fine scissors from the exact same direction that you are going to insert the catheter, because you need to have that little flap open to the catheter. **Once you've cut your cystic duct, you're dead.** Cholangiograms, common duct explorations, whatever—you're out of the ballgame for doing anything easily if you cut the duct.

Surgical Observations

Chief Resident

[1] Once the resident sees the 4-mm cystic duct, he or she correctly thinks back to the history to see if jaundice is present. Is there any evidence in the history for common duct obstruction?

Attending Surgeon

[2] The attending gives a brief account of how he would handle the large cystic duct. The patterns in his surgical scripts are better developed and stronger. He is not worried about a 4-mm cystic duct.

Judgment moderates the responses to recognized categories.

Cognitive Psychologist's Commentary: Laparoscopic Cholecystectomy

The attending did not consider the intraoperative finding of a 4-mm radiolucent defect anything to be concerned about. He would not do anything differently. The residents did not realize they could just leave it be, relying on the ERCP procedure to get rid of any stones that continued to be a problem postoperatively. As the attending observes, "Ninety percent of the stones pass, and 90% of those that don't can be handled by ERCP, so only 1% of the situations you don't handle will come back to you."

In this example, the knowledge of probabilities is used to put things into perspective. The residents know how to interpret the cholangiogram—it is most likely a stone. They also know the categories that apply to the situation: stones can happen, and stones can lead to various outcomes. And they know the available tools and their capabilities: postoperative ERCP and removal during the laparoscopic operation.

The difference is that the expert can use the basic categories with judgment. His knowledge that there is only about a 1% probability that the finding represents a problem informs his judgments of importance—the weights he gives to the possible positive or negative outcomes in the decision tree in his informal analysis. This knowledge, based on experience and discussion, is expressed as a probability estimate, but the probabilities may be more of a communication device than a reasoning tool.

The attending emphasized that his practice is constantly changing, not only because of new equipment and new techniques, but also because of changes in how much he trusts the gastroenterologists at his institution to do a ERCP to get rid of stones in the common duct.

36. JAUNDICE WITH PAIN

A 67-year-old man presents with vague epigastric pain of 2 weeks' duration. Subsequently he noticed gradual onset of jaundice with dark urine and clay-colored stools. He has had no previous abdominal surgery.

3rd-Year Resident

Let's start with a history and physical exam. I would ask if he has a history of gallstones or possibly a history of **alcohol abuse** or any stigmata related to alcohol consumption or abuse. Given the case description, I would then **look at laboratory data**, specifically his liver functions. Can you give me that information now? ☐

Chief Resident

First of all, I would do a standard history and physical examination with specific questions geared to potential malignancy, such as evidence of weight loss and so forth. I would also obtain laboratory values as a first step in assessing possible etiologies for the jaundice. That's about all I would do to start off.

Attending Surgeon

Sixty-seven years old? **This is a work-up of a patient with jaundice and some pain.** First of all, before I list my hypotheses, I'm going to do a physical exam to see if I can **feel a mass** in the abdomen and if the mass **feels like a gallbladder or a pancreatic cancer.**

I may even listen to the abdomen to see if I can hear a bruit over the splenic artery, which has been described in pancreatic cancer. I would take a history and find out if anything suggests hepatitis, such as a trip to Mexico, eating raw fish, a fondness for sushi, or whatever. I would call that out or have an internist do it. ☐

Then I would get some laboratory data. I would want to know his liver profile. It probably will not be helpful. His bilirubin will be elevated and the enzymes will be up a bit. There's a 50–50 chance that the liver profile will tell me something useful. **Hopefully the alk-phos will be extremely high, which will tip me off that the problem is obstructive jaundice.** Then I would get an **ultrasound** to see if there were stones in the gallbladder or if the ducts were dilated. But I always take what they say about the ducts with a grain of salt. Eventually, assuming that all of the evidence points toward obstructive jaundice, I would end up with an **ERCP.**

Endoscopy reveals a narrowing of the bile duct, measuring approximately 4 cm in length, extending from the bile duct just above the pancreas to above the entrance of the cystic duct into the common hepatic duct. CT scan reveals a normal liver except for dilated intrahepatic ducts. What would you do?

I'm concerned about the stricture of the common hepatic duct—it could be a malignancy. The patient has had no previous biliary tract surgery, right? So it's not an iatrogenic stricture, but it certainly could be malignancy.

At this point you need to stent him, to decompress the ducts. You could do it percutaneously with a transhepatic approach, or try to insert a stent with the ERCP and decompress the ducts. This may not succeed if he has proximal stricture. And the whole business of decompressing him may be controversial. It sounds like he needs a drainage procedure, such as a choledochojejunostomy, if it were amenable. The stricture may be proximal enough that he would require a hepaticojejunostomy, with an interhepatic stent procedure. Given this problem and what you've told me already, we have enough indications to proceed if the patient is an acceptable operative candidate. ☐

I would have ordered the ERCP and CT scan based on the laboratory findings. But given the fact that he has a narrow common duct from the pancreas to the cystic duct, I would obtain brushings from that area to look for any evidence of malignancy—by ERCP if possible. I would attempt to get a tissue diagnosis to elucidate what is going on. There's a possibility that the CT scan may be nondiagnostic and that further information can be obtained from an intraoperative procedure. ☐

We have a 4-cm stricture from the junction down into the full length of the common bile duct—I think that's what you're describing, right? And we haven't seen a mass in the pancreas on the CT or the ultrasound, and the liver looks okay.

A few weird thoughts crossed my mind. Common duct strictures can be associated with Crohn's disease and other funny things. But basically the patient is going to require an operation—an exploration of the common duct to see if there's a mass in the pancreas or anything abnormal about the common bile duct. If there's no mass in the pancreas, I would certainly open the common bile duct. You have to determine whether this is a stricture, sclerosing cholangitis, or tumor.

On exploration the patient is found to have firm pancratic head and prominent lymph nodes around the common bile duct. What now?

Again, you're concerned that he has cancer of the head of the pancreas. You'd like to make a diagnosis of that before embarking on a major procedure, such as a Whipple procedure. Sometimes that's not always possible to do. I would attempt to obtain biopsies, and I would use a transduodenal approach to avoid the complication of a pancreatic fistula. But I would attempt to get some tissue, which may not come back positive, from the mass in the head of the pancreas through a transduodenal approach.

First I would biopsy the lymph nodes as well as do a fine-needle aspiration of the end of the pancreas. That's what I would do first. ☐

That's good, because we can probably establish the diagnosis. The first thing is to harvest the node or nodes and send them for frozen section. If they are returned as tumor, then you finally know what you're dealing with. If they're benign, then you need to biopsy the pancreas, which I personally would probably do with a Travenol needle directly into the mass rather than transduodenally, although if I could get at the hard part of the mass transduodenally, I would do it. But the most important thing, if you can, is to establish a tissue diagnosis.

All node and pancreatic biopsies are negative.

3rd-Year Resident

You still don't know that you're not dealing with a malignancy. You can miss it and you're faced with a procedure such as a Whipple procedure or some type of decompressive procedure. Certainly this could represent pancreatitis from ductal obstruction. How old is the patient?

He is 67.

At this point I would forego the Whipple procedure and do a more proximal hepaticojejunostomy for decompression.

Chief Resident

At this point I think I would do a . . . (pause) The biopsies are negative for malignancy—what other information do they show?

Just negative.

Just negative. And once again the process on intraoperative evaluation involves the common duct from the cystic duct to the head of the pancreas. That's it? [4] (pause) Negative nodes are a fairly good sign. There is a possibility that this could be a benign disease. I probably would do a decompressive procedure. I think I would assess him, check the vessels to decide whether or not to do a Whipple procedure for benign disease or a decompressive procedure. I think I would probably assess him for resectability. I'd probably do a Whipple procedure. [5]

Attending Surgeon

You're in a really difficult situation—now you have to start thinking globally. With a 65-year-old man, you have to think about morbidity and mortality with surgery. You have to weigh the morbidity and the mortality of surgery.

I'd **open the common duct** and see if I can get any more information out of the common bile duct by either looking with the **scope** or biopsying. . . .

Biopsy shows adenocarcinoma of the wall of the common bile duct. Now what?

Do a Whipple.

Once again I'd assess him for resectability, for whether or not he would be able to tolerate a Whipple procedure as opposed to a simpler bypass procedure.

This is either a pancreatic tumor that has gone into the duct or a primary carcinoma of the duct. I would try to cure the patient, because some of these tumors are very slow growing. I would try to get high enough above the tumor, even if I had to cut both hepatic ducts separately and place them into a Roux-en-Y loop of bowel. I would resect the pancreas—Whipple procedure.

Surgical Observations

3rd-Year Resident

[1] The third-year resident is unaware that the laboratory data probably will not help in the management of this patient.

[2] The third-year resident has jumped to therapy before knowing the diagnosis. Whereas the attending tries to determine whether this is a stricture, sclerosing cholangitis, or something else, the resident thinks about the therapeutic options. The resident's thoughts are reasonable at this time, but an attempt to establish the diagnosis must be made simultaneously.

Chief Resident

[3] The chief resident prefers to do a fine-needle aspiration. The attending prefers a core-needle biopsy.

[4] The chief resident faces a mental block. He is trying to find out if the biopsy shows any information.

[5] The chief resident has jumped to doing a resection or a decompressive procedure, but he has let the diagnosis slip from his mind as a driving force. The attending would like to open the common bile duct to see what information about the diagnosis can be gathered there.

Attending Surgeon

[6] After his initial thoughts on the problem, the surgeon has "scanned" for zebras or other less frequent diseases that may cause a stricture of the common bile duct.

Experts use strategies for prolonging effective search when they are stuck for a diagnosis.

Cognitive Psychologist's Commentary: Jaundice with Pain

Strategies for allowing one's mind to work. In difficult problems the expert may not instantly recognize the best thing to do. It takes time to understand what is going on. Both the chief resident and the attending surgeon use strategies for buying a little time to think about this case.

The attending surgeon paused for several seconds after hearing the case description (the pause is not shown in the transcript). Then he repeated the key information that was presented: "67 years old? This is a work-up of a patient with jaundice and some pain" (after the initial presentation) and "We have a 4-cm stricture. . . . we haven't seen a mass in the pancreas . . . and the liver looks okay" (after the endoscopic report). These summaries are useful in that the presenter can correct him if he has heard incorrectly. But they have a more important role: repeating the key information keeps it in mind longer as a probe of the surgeon's long-term memory.[1] The process of interpreting what has been presented involves search through the memory for patterns that match, and the expert's two strategies, pausing and then repeating the key information, allow this search to go on longer and thus make it more likely that the surgeon will match the current situation with the most appropriate pattern he knows.

It is also useful to stimulate one's memory when making a decision. The chief resident's strategy can be seen in his thoughts after the biopsies come back negative. He paused a number of times after the unexpected negative biopsies and then began to weigh the alternatives—decompressing the duct or simply removing the whole thing with a Whipple procedure. During the time he was considering the alternatives, he stated that he would do each one. "I would probably do a decompressive procedure," he comments first, then later states, "I'd probably do a Whipple procedure." The chief resident's statements would sound indecisive to the casual listener, but we understand that he is "thinking aloud." In fact, his statements held up each option for his mind to react to, to judge whether it seemed right. This strategy is consistent with several of the recent, realistic models of the decision-making process, in which options are first evaluated wholistically for whether they seem right,[2] or at least better than the alternatives.[3] Only if there is doubt about which is best are the options analyzed in more detail.

Faced with the same surprising negative biopsies, the attending surgeon adopted a different tactic for buying time. He spoke very generally about the situation: "You're in a really difficult situation here. . . . This is a 65-year-old man, . . . you have to weigh the morbidity and mortality . . ." Then suddenly the tone of his voice shifted, and he announced, "I'd open the common duct." He had had an insight.[4]

The attending surgeon's strategy for buying time and letting his mind percolate may have advantages over the strategy adopted by the chief resident. The attending was not specific. He mentioned his general reaction to the situation, then he discussed broad considerations. Meantime, his mental search continued until suddenly it came up with an answer. The words he spoke did not sway the search process one way or the other. The chief resident, on the other hand, stated a series of specific ideas, focusing on the alternatives he was considering. This strategy did not give him much opportunity to come up with a third option, as the attending did. Furthermore, the chief resident's approach of asserting that he would do each option in turn involves a risk: if for some reason he were to be interrupted or could not let the comparison process continue until he had brought all his knowledge to bear, he might remember the last thing he said— "I would probably do a decompressive procedure"—as a final decision rather than as a step in his evaluation of the options.

The attending surgeon's general comments, when he was blocked and casting about, use the vocabulary of a general decision analysis: "Be sure to consider the mortality and morbidity of each of the options." A decision analysis would go on to specify the dimensions of morbidity that need to be considered and to devise procedures for measuring them and trading them off against mortality and against the possible gains of the procedures.[5] But here the surgeon used these ideas just as a filler, as an orienting device to help him continue to think about the problem while his automatic processes of pattern recognition worked. In addition, mentioning the ideas may have activated related concepts in the mental network of his knowledge, making it more likely that the final insight would spare the patient pain or risk of death.

1. Abernathy CM, Hamm RM: Surgical Intuition. Philadelphia, PA, Hanley & Belfus, 1994, chapter 3.
2. Mitchell TR, Beach LR: "Do I love thee? Let me count. . ." Toward an understanding of intuitive and automatic decision making. Organiz Behav Hum Decision Making, 47:1–20, 1990.
3. Montgomery H: From cognition to action: The search for dominance in decision making. In Montgomery H, Svenson O (eds): Process and Structure in Human Decision Making. New York, Wiley, 1989, pp 23–49.
4. Abernathy CM, Hamm RM: Surgical Intuition. Philadelphia, PA, Hanley & Belfus, 1994, chapter 9.
5. Abernathy CM, Hamm RM: Surgical Intuition. Philadelphia, PA, Hanley & Belfus, 1994, chapter 7.

37. EPIGASTRIC PAIN

A 28-year-old man presents to the ED complaining of epigastric pain. He is a known consumer of alcohol and has no other significant medical history. He has a temperature on admission of 39°C.

1st-Year Resident

If it's predominantly gastric pain, then you could think of peptic ulcer disease, cholecystitis, or some sort of biliary disease. In a known alcohol abuser you may also want to think of pancreatitis, especially in someone who's 28. Did you tell me his white blood cell count? Just that his temperature is elevated? You can also think of gastroenteritis. You want **some laboratory tests** to see whether or not he has an elevated amylase. That would be a nonspecific indicator that something was going on intraabdominally: if he has a huge elevation of his **amylase**, you'd think harder about pancreatitis. You can check his **liver enzymes** to see whether or not he has evidence of biliary obstruction.

3rd-Year Resident

The differential diagnosis includes gallstones and pancreatitis, especially with an alcoholic. You need studies of liver function. On the physical exam, I want to see **just how tender he is.** A rigid abdomen is a fairly classic sign of a perforated ulcer, and you want to go right to the operating room. If the exam isn't remarkable, you want more studies to figure out what's going on: CBC chemistries including amylase (LFTs) and **ultrasound of the gallbladder.**

Attending Surgeon

I want to **examine the abdomen to see if in fact he has peritoneal signs.** I want to do a few things to see where the fever is coming from, including a chest x-ray and a white count just to corroborate that. I would get a **3-way chest x-ray** to see if there is any **free air,** to see if there is any **bowel obstruction.** I would take a history of aspirin ingestion or other barrier breakers. ☐

He has a white blood cell count of 25,000; amylase that is high-normal; LFTs that are elevated with bilirubin of 4 and SGOT of 350; and a left shift in his white blood cell count. You are asked to come back to the ED an hour later because he is hypotensive.

I would start IV fluids to stabilize his blood pressure. I want to know his hematocrit, to see whether or not I may be tempted to think that he was bleeding acutely from something. You may want to know whether his elevated liver enzymes and elevated bilirubin are direct or indirect. Then you could differentiate whether or not the problem is obstructive. Get some lab work. Definitely resuscitate him.

That sounds bad. It really doesn't rule out any of the possibilities. Obviously, you've got to resuscitate him right away, with lots of fluids. Probably he needs to go to OR or at least the intensive care unit for resuscitation.

I would start an IV and give him some fluids. I would get an ultrasound of his gallbladder and pancreas and see if they can visualize the common duct. ☑ I might draw blood for some more sophisticated hepatitis screening. I might think about getting a CT exam.

Surgical Observations

[1] Notice the contrast in the use of the radiology department for this patient. Radiology has become extremely important in making surgical diagnoses. Notice, however, that the first-year resident does not use radiology at all, the second-year resident uses radiology for a gallbladder ultrasound, and the attending surgeon uses it for a 3-way radiograph of the abdomen. At this stage, knowing which area to look at becomes the critical point of the work-up of the patient.

[2] Contrast the approaches of the first-year resident and the attending surgeon to the work-up of the bilirubin of 4. The first-year resident orders a direct vs. indirect bilirubin (of minimal to no value), whereas the attending surgeon orders an ultrasound of the gallbladder, pancreas, and common duct.

Rigid structure helps residents to learn scripts.

Cognitive Psychologist's Commentary: Epigastric Pain

One important difference among doctors with different levels of experience is the importance of the physical exam. The attending surgeon says immediately, "I want to examine the abdomen." The third-year resident lays out a brief list of possible hypotheses, mentions liver function tests, and then expresses his intention to "see just how tender" the abdomen is. But the first-year resident never gets to the physical exam. He talks at length about hypotheses, gathering pertinent information, and possible actions, and what he says is generally consistent with what the third-year resident and the attending say.

Unlike the first-year resident in the think-aloud about Left Lower Quadrant Pain (p. 166), who was either too shy to talk or did not yet have the required structure, this first-year resident has much to say about this paper patient. His thoughts are guided by a structured framework that is the basic cognitive tool that he will develop, over the years, into the expert's automated pattern recognition capability. The third-year resident also has such a framework. For example, he says the name of one of the categories in which he organizes his knowledge: physical exam. This organized structure serves the residents in several ways.[1] For example, this familiar mental structure provides rapid access to the appropriate knowledge that the doctor needs to understand what is going on with a patient. By going over the same sorts of ideas and questions in the same order with every patient, the resident is building up a large chunk of knowledge that can come rapidly to mind. However, he does not want this structure to become too automatic right away, because it is not yet correct or complete.

The first-year resident's medical knowledge, organized in the basic framework of the patient encounter, is quite correct in some spots. It enabled the resident to propose a list of likely hypotheses and to name tests that could be used to support or eliminate those hypotheses. His hypotheses were in the right ballpark: he mentioned five hypotheses, the third-year resident mentioned four, and the attending mentioned none specifically (although hypotheses are, of course, implicit in the tests he considers as he "works forward"[2]). The hyopthesis list of the third-year resident and attending are subsets of the first-year resident's list. Another sign of the first-year resident's knowledge is that he anticipated the tests that were reported by the presenter of the case in the second paragraph.

But the first-year resident's knowledge structure is deficient in three ways: (1) it is incomplete, (2) it is incorrect, and (3) it does not suggest ideas according to how important they are likely to be. The task of the resident and his or her teachers is to correct or tune the knowledge structure[3,4] in detail—to make it complete as well as correct and to support the doctor's judgments of what is most important in each situation.[4] The exposure of the resident's current ideas is essential for this tuning process. Because people do not learn simply from passive exposure to situations that are different from their current knowledge, they must (1) have the correct representation of the situation actively in mind and (2) embed it in their knowledge so that next time the new, correct representation comes to mind.

Having a structured way of understanding patients that is used for every patient allows the required learning. The fact that the resident will "go through it the same way every time" means that the same representation (or part of his or her knowledge base) will be made active when a similar patient is encountered. Within this framework, the resident will acquire more and more medical facts, available when they are needed because of their position in the structural organization that is activated when the situation calls for it.

This process is useful not only for acquiring new ideas but also for correcting ideas that are already in place. The particular facts mounted in the framework receive feedback from various sources, and the feedback affects how likely they are to be used again.

One source of feedback is what actually happens with patients. The resident will eventually stop considering a disease category that he or she never encounters, such as porphyria. And a few surprises will make a missed diagnosis come very easily to mind when it is appropriate. Anderson and Schooler[3] have described the ability of human memory to recall ideas according to the frequency with which they have been encountered in the past. This feature, which underlies quick recognition of the familiar, makes human memory optimal when all ideas are of about equal value. However, doctors also need to be on the lookout for diseases that they may have rarely or never seen, particularly those that have terrible consequences if not quickly recognized and treated. Thus the doctor's knowledge needs inputs other than his or her own experience.

The second source of feedback is comparison with what others think. When residents hear a peer or someone with more experience talk about a case or they read the think-alouds of expert surgeons, they gain another source for fleshing out or trimming their own facts.

A third source is explicit instruction, as when the attending says, "In this sort of case, you should think of ruptured abdominal aortic aneurysm," or "You don't need to think of black widow spider bites; when you hear hoofbeats, don't think of zebras." Here the instructor can provide the required knowledge directly.[6]

As a fourth source of feedback, the medical knowledge that the resident is building up within the framework, already visible in this case, can be specifically criticized. Residents' thinking is corrected and critiqued at case presentations or on rounds. "What did you think of? What else should you have thought of? Why was that test irrelevant, given what you already knew?" This is the function of the objective review.[7]

The sources of feedback and correction of the resident's knowledge, beyond simple exposure to many cases, eventually allow the doctor to judge rapidly what is most important to do for a patient.

1. Abernathy CM, Hamm RM: Surgical Intuition. Philadelphia, PA, Hanley & Belfus, 1994, chapters 3 and 4.
2. Patel VL, Groen GJ, Norman GR: Effects of conventional and problem-based medical curricula on problem solving. Acad Med 66:380–389, 1991.
3. Anderson JR, Schooler LJ: Reflections of the environment in memory. Psycyhol Sci 2:396–408, 1991.
4. Schwartz S, Griffin T: Medical Thinking: The Psychology of Medical Judgment and Decision Making. New York, Springer-Verlag, 1986, chapter 5.
5. Dreyfus HL, Dreyfus SE: Mind over Machine: The Power of Human Intuition and Expertise in the Era of the Computer. New York, The Free Press, 1986.
6. Johnson-Laird PN: The Computer and the Mind: An Introduction to Cognitive Science. Cambridge, MA, Harvard University Press, 1988, chapter 7.
7. Abernathy CM, Hamm RM: Surgical Intuition. Philadelphia, PA, Hanley & Belfus, 1994, chapters 5 and 11.

38.   ABDOMINAL AORTIC ANEURYSM

A 64-year-old obese man, who is a known alcoholic, presents to the ED with a 2-hour history of severe epigastric abdominal pain. His BP is 200/110, HR is 110 bpm, and his stool is trace hematest-positive.

1st-Year Resident

My first concern is what brought him in. That is what I want to address initially, just to make sure that I know the facts. I am very concerned about his abdominal pain and about his blood pressure. I am worried that he has intraabdominal bleeding of some kind. I would like to know how long he's had the abdominal pain.

3rd-Year Resident

First of all, you have to establish IV lines and instigate resuscitation ☐ with fluid. Then you begin your investigation to determine the nature of his abdominal pain. Basic laboratory tests should be ordered: chest x-ray, KUB. Specifically, you entertain diagnoses such as duodenal ulcer, perforated or not, some sort of gastric problem, problems associated with the history of alcoholism and potentially a history of blood clots.

5th-Year Resident

I first thought of ulcer disease or some other alcohol-related duodenal or gastric process, but in the back of my mind I think that **I need to rule out something separate from the alcohol disease, like an abdominal aortic aneurysm**—especially in view of the belly pain. With the trace hematest-positive stool, I think of ulcers ☐ and something going along with that. I want to know if he has been vomiting and what that would show. I would like to get more information about related symptoms.

Attending Surgeon

Obese, alcoholic male with epigastric pain, hematest-positive stool from below. I am going to start IVs and get some baseline laboratory data—CBC, maybe a 3-way radiograph of the abdomen. I certainly want a hematocrit to see whether he has really lost a significant amount of blood ☐ and maybe baseline liver function tests and a chest x-ray. **I am thinking, "epigastric pain in an alcoholic male: gastritis, perforated ulcer."** Biliary tract is unlikely.

Laboratory tests are ordered in the ED. The patient has a hematocrit of 38, an arterial PO$_2$ of 7.25, a PCO$_2$ of 80, and a base deficit of 10. Abdominal ultrasound in the ED is nondiagnostic because of too much gas. His EKG shows sinus tachycardia, his bilirubin is 0.7, his alkaline phosphatase is 100, his SGOT is 37, his BP is 100/P, and his HR is 120.

The patient is acidotic, and so far that is the only abnormal test result I know about. His

Clearly we have not established a diagnosis yet. I am not able to ask for specific answers to test results.

Actually it sounds like a perforated duodenal ulcer with the abdominal pain. I would like to know what his

His hematocrit is 38 or thereabouts, and his blood pressure has dropped. I got no information from the 3-way blood pressure is dropping, and I am still very concerned about abdominal bleeding. [3]

The patient is acidotic, his BP continues to drop, and he is becoming more tachycardic despite resuscitation. Therefore, I would consider some sort of intraabdominal catastrophe. [3] I still think that he may have a perforated duodenal ulcer or some other abdominal problem. Was there anything on chest x-ray or KUB—free air or anything like that? A few critical pieces of information are missing.

belly feels like, and I would have done a physical exam before I ordered the tests. If he had a rigid abdomen, all of that could have been circumvented. You are saying that he is acidotic, and he is going into shock. On the basis of the hematocrit, he is not a big GI bleeder.

radiograph—that bothers me. I would do an **abdominal exam** to see if he is tender anywhere. I would put in an **NG tube** to see if I can ascertain that we are really dealing with upper GI bleeding. It is possible it can even be lower GI. Pain plus drop in BP might mean ruptured aneurysm. CT would help—or that 3-way. I do not think upper GI endoscopy is going to help. I put in the NG tube first to see if there is any blood.

Thirty minutes later you have administered a bolus of lactated Ringer's solution and started an IV of 150 cc/hr. His BP now is 110, his HR is 110, and his CT scan shows a 6-cm abdominal aortic aneurysm with a 4-cm iliac aneurysm, along with fluid in the pelvis.

The concern is certainly the fluid and whether or not the aneurysms have ruptured slightly and are bleeding. An aneurysm of that size, if it has not ruptured, has a 50% or so chance of rupture within the next few years. He definitely **needs an operation.**

You have established that he has an aneurysm and fluid in his pelvis. You need to **take him to the operating room** after he has been adequately resuscitated. [4]

So actually this was leading toward an abdominal aortic aneurysm. It sounds like he is leaking, and hypotensive—it sounds like we are **going to have to operate.**

He definitely responded to the fluids, so it was hypovolemia. I think the aneurysm is significant. I need another hematocrit. I guess a couple of hours have passed. We are going to insert a Swan-Ganz catheter and do all the stuff for volume to nail down that it was hypovolemia. I need to know whether the CT showed any retroperitoneal hematoma. **I do not think we have too much time to mess around**—we are moving to the OR. Ultrasound is not going to give any more information than the CT did. I would love to know if the fluid in the pelvis is blood rather than ascites or something else. I am going to assume it probably is blood. I might even do a DPL to find out. If the DPL is positive, **we are heading to the OR.**

Surgical Observations

[1] The third-year resident decides to give IV fluids for resuscitation in a patient with a BP of 200/110 and a HR of 110. On the basis of this information alone, it is difficult to determine that resuscitation should be part of the initial plan. Neither the fifth-year nor the attending is concerned about "resuscitation," although both used IVs.

[2] The attending puts little if any importance on the "trace hematest-positive stool." The fifth-year resident, on the other hand, lets the test lead him toward thinking about blood loss from ulcers. The attending is able to ignore the test, which is typical of many tests in medicine—that is, it has very high sensitivity and very low specificity.

[3] The first-year resident uses the term "abdominal bleeding," which does not help him to focus on whether the bleeding is retroperitoneal, intraperitoneal, or gastrointestinal. The third-year resident uses the term "intraabdominal catastrophe," which is probably a better term in this instance, because it is not clear that the problem is blood loss. It could be a perforated viscus, among other possibilities.

[4] "Adequately resuscitating" a ruptured abdominal aortic aneurysm may not be possible or desirable before going to the OR.

With experience, surgeons rely on more specific maxims.

Cognitive Psychologist's Commentary: Abdominal Aortic Aneurysm

This set of think-alouds, by surgeons at four levels of experience, makes it very easy to see the progression in the ideas that the surgeons bring to the case. We can see differences in what the surgeons recognize and in the strategies they use.

The ideas that come to mind become both more detailed and more focused as one gains experience. Consider what the surgeons saw in the case description and its connection to their diagnostic hypotheses. The first-year resident, who saw abdominal pain and high blood pressure, worried about intraabdominal bleeding. This, of course, is correct but nonspecific. The others show more specific ideas. They look for particular observations or test results and have more specific explanations for the patient's symptoms. The first-year resident is still trying to figure out what to notice, whereas the more experienced residents usually notice the right facts but still have to figure out what to do with them.

Both the fifth-year resident and the attending surgeon considered the possibility of abdominal aortic aneurysm before it was reported in the CT scan results. They mentioned it at different times. The fifth-year resident mentioned it after the first description of the patient as part of his broad initial response. The attending surgeon mentioned it after receiving the laboratory tests and hearing of the sudden drop in blood pressure. For the fifth-year resident, it was a general rule: "If an alcoholic presents with belly pain, rule out abdominal aortic aneurysm before assuming ulcer." For the attending, it was a more specific recognition: "Pain plus drop in blood pressure may mean ruptured aneurysm." The difference between the two is a sign of "tuning" one's knowledge.[1] The attending's mind works more efficiently, applying hypotheses when they are most likely to be needed, not bothering to consider them explicitly when there is not yet sufficient reason.

When you don't have a well-tuned script that enables you to recognize automatically the key features of the situation, to identify the important hypotheses, and to respond appropriately, you have to figure out the situation logically. In this kind of problem solving, rules of thumb can be helpful.[2] As one gains experience, the rules become more specific, as befits more specific knowledge.

Thus, the first-year resident guides his thinking with a very general rule: "Pay attention to what brought the patient in." It orients him to the need to find out all the facts, yet not to become distracted by aspects of the patient's history that are unrelated to the present illness. The fifth-year resident also uses a rule: "Don't get fooled by the most obvious hypothesis," which reminds him to keep other hypotheses in mind and to look for opportunities to rule them out. Even though this general rule[3,4] helped him to state the correct hypothesis of abdominal aortic aneurysm early in his thinking, the observation of the drop in blood pressure did not return his attention to it. At that point[3,4] the attending recognized the correct hypothesis, although he had not explicitly put it on his initial list.

---

1. Abernathy CM, Hamm RM: Surgical Intuition. Philadelphia, PA, Hanley & Belfus, 1994, chapter 4.
2. Bursztajn H, Hamm RM: Medical maxims: Two views of science. Yale J Biol Med 52:483–486, 1979.
3. Perkins DN, Salomon G: Are cognitive skills context-bound? Educ Res 18(1):16–25, 1989.
4. Abernathy CM, Hamm RM: Surgical Intuition. Philadelphia, PA, Hanley & Belfus, 1994, chapter 5.

39. LEFT LOWER QUADRANT PAIN

A 57-year-old man comes to the emergency department. He has had 2 days of left lower-quadrant abdominal pain and what he thought was a low-grade fever. WBC is 12.5, his temperature is 38.5° C, and the left lower quadrant is tender. You put him in the hospital. What are your thoughts about the patient?

1st-Year Resident

I have already examined him and taken a history. I would get a belly film to see what that showed, **acquire a stool sample to see if he is bleeding**, and make sure that he is stable.

3rd-Year Resident

I would start with his history to see whether he has had any similar attacks before, any abdominal pain, any abdominal surgery, or symptoms that he hasn't been able to describe well, like diarrhea or change in bowel habits. I'd examine him to get an idea of how tender he is and do a rectal exam to make sure he is not bleeding from below. In a 55-year-old man, especially with abdominal pain on the left side, you wonder about diverticulitis. I'd want a **3-way radiograph of the abdomen**, see if he has normal gas patterns or if there is any perforation **(free air)**—anything that would make me go to the OR emergently. Beyond that I would admit him and put him on IV antibiotics to make sure he gets fluids and is well hydrated. You may have to operate acutely.

Attending Surgeon

The first things that cross my mind are perforated diverticulitis, cancer, ischemic colitis—a kind of broad differential diagnosis. The first step I think is general resuscitation more than anything else. I would assess fluids, urine output, and acid-base balance. Then an early decision needs to be made about whether or not he should go to the OR. **Peritoneal findings would shift me toward wanting to explore him** if I felt he was clinically stable. At that point I'd be inclined to get a CT of the abdomen. ②

On day 1 you get a CT scan. His temperature is still 38.5° C, and he still has the same abdominal pain and tenderness. CT scan shows edema of the left colon wall.

That's all? If I have not taken **blood cultures**, I would do that. I would probably at least consider an endoscopy. ①

The CT scan tells me that the problem is the colon. It could still be diverticulitis, ischemia, colitis, diarrhea, or anything like that.

At this point I would think that the overall picture is consistent with diverticular disease or ischemic colitis. **I would be interested in his physical exam** at this point. ③

His fever mounts to between 38.5° and 39° C every day. On day 5 his blood count rises to 16,000. He is still tender in the lower left quadrant.

1st-Year Resident	3rd-Year Resident	Attending Surgeon
I would probably consider repeating the **CT exam.** I'd check the belly exam and make sure that it hasn't changed.	You could **scope him** to look for anything that would sway you from operating, but at that point you are still concerned that he has an abscess and needs an operation.	At this point I think that **the patient has failed conservative therapy.**[4]

Surgical Observations

1st-Year Resident

[1] The first year resident has not made the negative connection between diverticulitis and colonic endoscopy. That is, colonoscopy and sigmoidoscopy are of minimal to no value in the diagnosis of diverticulitis. Knowing the *non*-value of a test or exam may have as much importance as knowing the value.

Attending Surgeon

[2] Note that of the three surgeons, the attending surgeon emphasizes the peritoneal findings (a physical finding), whereas the other two emphasize x-ray. The third-year resident would go to the OR if there were "free air" on the 3-way radiograph, and the first-year resident acquired a stool sample to see if there was bleeding.

[3] Once again, the attending surgeon has emphasized the physical exam and constantly comes back to it as the critical factor.

[4] The attending surgeon is comfortable with the decision to go to the OR. At this point, the third-year resident is beginning to come to that decision, but he still flirts with ideas like endoscopy or other things that will "keep us out of the OR."

The structured knowledge of the expert is organized for action.

Cognitive Psychologist's Commentary: Left Lower Quadrant Pain

Remarkable here are the differences among the doctors' responses to the same case, which are a function of their levels of experience. The first-year resident has a rudimentary response, naming a few tests and emphasizing the important goal of assuring the patient's stability. He shows little evidence of understanding what is, or could be, going on and mentions no specific hypotheses about possible causes of the left lower-quadrant pain. In particular, he seems to have no conception of what may require an operation.

The first-year resident knows the general script: he already would have examined the patient and taken a history. But he does not know what to expect, what the likely findings of the examination and history would have been, or where the findings would have taken him. Of course, this first-year resident would recognize the hypotheses and responses of the others, and, if given 15 minutes to think about it, probably could have produced a respectable list of possible causes and appropriate responses. But this information was not available to his mind immediately on hearing the description of the case. The first-year resident's knowledge is not yet organized to provide instant recognition, that is, rapid access to the needed information, either in the form of an illness script or a recalled case.[1]

The third-year resident shows a comprehensive and structured response to the case, exceeding not only the first-year resident but also the attending in the number of detailed hypotheses and possible tests. The attending, in contrast, focuses on what is important: the two primary diagnostic candidates, the need for resuscitation, and the need to consider whether an immediate operation is required. The third-year resident reaches the same points eventually but includes ideas that the attending did not consider worth mentioning. Because any hypothesis can trigger a test, the generation of numerous hypotheses increases the chances of iatrogenic harm.[2] In addition, Lesgold[3] has observed that residents at intermediate levels of training may actually do worse than either novices or experts (see box below).

**Not all learning is monotonic:
sometimes practice produces worse performance.**

Lesgold reported the following results of his study of resident radiologists (amount of experience: 10,000 x-rays) and senior hospital staff (experience: 500,000 x-rays):

> We gave them some very difficult cases to solve and analyzed their diagnoses, their defense of their diagnoses, their ability to incorporate new evidence (laboratory test data) into diagnoses to which they were already committed, and even their ability to outline, on the x-ray film, the abnormalities they claimed to see.[4]

> On some cases, new residents did almost as well as senior staff and better than third- and fourth-year residents. In fact, in a few cases the same person, looking at the same film, made the correct diagnosis in his first year but the wrong one in his third year. When we examined this result in detail, it became apparent that the new residents had been successful initially because the films were classic, almost textbook examples of particular diseases. Such films can be tricky, because the basic features that stand out, although classic indicators of one disease, may also be consistent with several others. New residents seemed to have little ability to consider critically the less likely alternatives, so they made the most likely choice. After additional training, they knew that the alternatives had to be considered, but they still did not have the capability of choosing definitively among them. As a result, they sometimes chose a less likely alternative that they did not know enough to rule out.[5]

The attending organizes his thoughts around the key decision: "An early decision needs to be made as to whether or not he should go to the OR." The third-year resident's thoughts, on the other hand, dwell longer within the generic structure of the diagnostic patient encounter: "What conditions do I suspect, what tests would I do, what questions would I ask?"

With experience, the expert has developed an organized body of knowledge that is both complete and automatically accessible. The third-year resident shows an intermediate developmental stage in this process: knowledge that is well structured and rich but does not yet rapidly and automatically focus on the most important aspects of the situation. The automaticity comes with many repeated responses to similar situations, and the correctness of the automatic response depends on whether the resident has engaged in deliberate consideration many times along the way.

We see evidence of such deliberation around the decision whether to go to the OR after the developments (such as increased WBC) on the fifth day. At this point the attending immediately concludes that conservative therapy has failed and that it is time to go to the OR. The third-year resident recognizes the same conclusion, but also questions himself to check whether that decision is correct. Such checking, done habitually, keeps the resident's knowledge and practice correct while they are slowly becoming automatic through repeated use.[6]

Given this context, it would be silly for a resident to try to emulate the expert by making momentous decisions quickly and without checking. Such shooting from the hip would probably produce errors at an unacceptable rate. Of course, individuals vary in degree of cautiousness: some will obsessively review their first responses for years after the accurate response has become automatic, whereas others have to be told to slow down and to think it out.

In the first-year resident the knowledge structure, organized for response to patients, is only nascent. Of interest, the elements that appear are the essential backbone of what is to come, including references to the physical exam and history and to procedures for looking closer. In the actual situation, the results of these actions would trigger other responses in the first-year resident, hopefully leading in the right direction. In addition, the first-year resident pays attention to the immediate needs of the patient, that is, his clinical stability. All these elements are mentioned, more elaborately, by both more experienced physicians.

1. Schmidt HG, Norman GR, Boshuizen HPA: A cognitive perspective on medical expertise: Theory and implications. Acad Med 65:611–621, 1990.
2. Mold JW, Stein HF: The cascade effect in the clinical care of patients. N Engl J Med 314:512–514, 1986.
3. Lesgold A: Problem solving. In Sternberg RJ, Smith EE (eds): The Psychology of Human Thought. New York, Cambridge University Press, 1988, pp 188–213.
4. Lesgold, p 202.
5. Lesgold, pp 203–204.
6. Abernathy CM, Hamm RM: Surgical Intuition. Philadelphia, PA, Hanley & Belfus, 1994, chapter 4.

40. SMALL BOWEL OBSTRUCTION

A 45-year-old woman presents with abdominal pain and vomiting. The pain awoke her at 4:00 a.m. and has persisted throughout the day. You see her at 4:00 p.m. in the ED. She had a hysterectomy 5 years ago and is otherwise healthy. Basic lab tests are normal. A 3-way radiograph of the abdomen shows what the radiology resident calls a small bowel obstruction. What else do you want to ask the patient? How do you want to manage her?

3rd-Year Resident

Her abdominal pain began at 4:00 in the morning. Has she been throwing up? Does she have a fever? When was her last bowel movement? Is she passing gas? Are the symptoms worsening? I would place a nasogastric tube to see what kind of output I have from that. You said that basic laboratory tests were normal. I assume that includes a white blood cell count. Depending on the results I receive from all those things, I would get an upper GI, with a **small bowel follow-through.** ☐

5th-Year Resident

I would get a bit more **history** from the patient: whether this is the first occurrence of this type of abdominal pain, where the pain is located, and the characteristic nature of the pain. Is it crampy pain, continuous pain, sharp pain? Does it radiate? I would ask her about the nature of her vomiting. Is it bilious? Is it bloody? I would find out when her last bowel movement was and whether she has been passing any flatus. I would ask about other symptoms. Does she have dysuria, diarrhea, or any other recent medical problems, such as the flu, cough, or fevers? I would ask about her previous surgery. She had a hysterectomy. Did they make an incision in her abdomen? Did it go up and down or across? Did they do anything else when they took out her uterus, such as remove her appendix?

Attending Surgeon

I want to know if the patient has had any episodes like this before. I want to examine her for any external evidence of inguinal **hernias,** femoral hernias, or obturator hernias. I would include a pelvic exam. I suppose **I would ask her if she has any idea about what caused the symptoms.** Did she swallow a peach pit or persimmon pit or experience any trauma? I would ask other historical questions about abdominal pain. Did they take out her appendix when she had the hysterectomy? Are her ovaries still intact? Is the pain steady or crampy? That will do for starters.

When you review the x-ray yourself, you notice gas in the colon. The patient tells you she has been passing gas intermittently. What do you do?

It is a partial obstruction. In that case, I would admit her for IV hydration and

At this point, it is still possible that she has a bowel obstruction—it could be a partial obstruction. I want to

Gas in the colon to me does not necessarily mean that she does not have a small bowel

bowel rest to prevent it from progressing to a complete obstruction. Again, I would obtain a small bowel followthrough.

You insert a nasogastric tube and watch her overnight. The following morning, the patient is no better, but she has less pain. The NG tube has produced 1200 cc overnight. At this stage, what clinical parameters would help you to decide whether to operate? What would make you not operate?

On physical exam, you said she feels better, but her abdomen is tender and that there is quite a bit of output from the nasogastric tube. I would go mostly on the physical exam.

make sure that this is not an ileus that is being misinterpreted and that she does not have other pathology. At this point the abdominal exam would be important to see if she had any localized tenderness or peritoneal signs. I would look at the film carefully to see if she had any evidence of free air in the abdomen, which would suggest perforated viscus. I would make sure she did not have any air in her biliary tree on the film. The abdominal exam would direct me at this point. [2]

The four classic factors that we look for in patients with small bowel obstruction are **fever, tachycardia, leukocytosis, or abdominal tenderness.** If she had any of those signs and has failed a period of conservative management, I would operate. [3] The other alternative is to give her contrast through the NG tube into the small bowel followthrough to see if she indeed has a complete obstruction.

obstruction because the gas could have been there before the obstruction or she could have a little bit of gas going through into her colon. I do not worry about that too much in making the diagnosis. I would probably insert an **NG tube.** If she is not toxic or septic, with no elevated white count and no fever, I would reexamine her and see what happens.

I would repeat the 3-way radiograph of the abdomen, **focusing specifically on what had happened to the size of the small bowel.** If the small bowel was moderately to largely dilated and had either stayed that way or become larger, I would operate. If the size of the small bowel had become smaller with fewer loops and it looked like the problem may be resolving, I may try another day or two of NG suction. If her white blood cell count or her fever was up or if I thought she was sick with it (patients usually are not), that would make me operate. But fundamentally, I would go on the basis of the 3-way radiograph of the abdomen. [4]

Surgical Observations

3rd-Year Resident

[1] The small bowel study is a good idea. More often than not, it helps to define the situation.

5th-Year Resident

[2] The physical examination in small bowel obstruction, except for excluding external hernias or eliciting the abdominal tenderness of dead bowel (note the mild abdominal tenderness), is not among the strong "trigger" pieces of data.

[3] The fifth-year resident realizes that there are two reasons to operate on a small bowel obstruction in this setting: failed conservative therapy and a combination of signs that suggest dead bowel. The fifth-year resident (like most fifth-year residents) tends to emphasize the dead-bowel indication for operation. In fact, most patients do not have dead bowel, but they fail conservative therapy. Thus it really is the failure of conservative therapy that drives most decisions to operate on a small bowel obstruction.

Attending Surgeon

[4] The clearest difference in management is the attending surgeon's lesser concern about ischemic bowel and greater concern for making an early, accurate decision about the possibility of spontaneous resolution of the small bowel obstruction. The attending surgeon has a much lower expectation of dead bowel than either of the residents, who have dead bowel (the most serious complication) as their prime thought. Through case experience the attending surgeon diluted that concern. For the attending, there are two indications to operate: (1) unresolved small bowel obstruction or (2) signs or symptoms of ischemic small bowel. In his experience, he has responded to the first indication earlier and more frequently; he rarely operates on the basis of the second indication. Thus, if the obstruction appears "set" (based on small bowel diameter with no further gas in colon and so forth), the patient requires early operation; this obviates any concern for discovering ischemic bowel before the operation. The attending frequently has been bailed out by operating earlier, but for unresolved small bowel obstruction rather than for the presence of ischemic bowel.

The expert surgeon visualizes the patient's anatomy.

Cognitive Psychologist's Commentary:
Small Bowel Obstruction

In their scripts for thinking about small bowel obstruction, the more experienced surgeons use their knowledge of anatomy more than the third-year resident. Although they do not get to see the patient or to view films, they indicate specific signs and symptoms that they would be looking for. In addition, visual thinking plays a more central role in their use of information.[1]

After receiving the first description of the patient in the ED, the attending surgeon is interested in the history of previous operations. Were her appendix and/or her ovaries removed? The chief resident also asks what other organs may have been removed as well as about the orientation of the incision. The third-year resident did not consider this type of information.

In trying to understand the source of the patient's abdominal pain, the experienced surgeon frequently tries to visualize what is going on internally. Knowledge about the location of previous operations and general knowledge about the effects of adhesions contribute to the surgeon's mental representation of the patient's abdomen; that is, the surgeon may actually construct a specific mental image of the patient's organs and correlate it with the external appearance, with how the patient reacts when various parts of the abdomen are palpated, and with the x-ray images.

After the description of the patient's condition the following morning, the surgeon's thoughts about whether to operate reveal additional differences in his use of visual information. The third-year resident says that she would go mainly on the basis of the exam. The fifth-year resident is a little more specific, citing four signs that would prove small bowel obstruction and require operation if the obstruction doesn't resolve with conservative management. He also mentions that an x-ray would be useful but does not specify how. The attending says that a repeat 3-way radiograph of the abdomen would drive his decision.

As noted in the surgical observations, the residents are primarily concerned about the possibility that the bowel may be dead, whereas the attending focuses on whether the obstruction looks like it will resolve, dead or not. Perhaps because of this different focus, but mainly because of his greater use of visualization, the attending is much more explicit about the use of the x-ray information: he would look at the change in the size of the bowel. Again, the attending seeks visual information for his visual representation of the patient's abdomen.

Studies of how expert radiologists differ from novices show that they build a thorough representation of the patient's anatomy. They "spend proportionately more of their problem-solving time generating a representation of the situation. . . . When they talk about an x-ray film, they use more anatomy terms and speak in greater detail. . . . They also have more elaborate general plans for dealing with different types of disease situations that enable them to describe more precisely the situation that seems to be present."[2] These characteristics are evident in the attending surgeon's thoughts, even in the absence of an actual x-ray image.

---

1. Abernathy CM, Hamm RM: Surgical Intuition. Philadelphia, PA, Hanley & Belfus, 1994, chapter 10.
2. Lesgold A: Problem solving. In Sternberg RJ, Smith EE (eds): The Psychology of Human Thought. New York, Cambridge University Press, 1988, p 203.

41. PELVIC FRACTURE

You are called to the ED to see a 35-year-old woman who was the unrestrained driver in a motor vehicle accident involving moderate speed but unknown direction of force. The staff have examined her; pulse is 130, BP is 115/80, hematocrit is 35. Physical exam reveals no external evidence of trauma and no findings except a probable pelvic fracture.

1st-Year Resident

The history and physical exam so far sound fairly thorough. You're ready for the secondary review. I'm still worried because the patient is tachycardic, so I would ask her about past medical problems and things like that as well as begin the usual IV resuscitation.

3rd-Year Resident

I would treat it as a serious high mechanism injury and get large-bore access—all the standard stuff—proceed to x-ray survey, with early DPL. If she is grossly positive on DPL, she would go straight to the OR. If she were anything else, we would treat her conservatively if it turns out that she has a pelvic fracture. [2]

Attending Surgeon

[Both paragraphs were read to the attending at once. The response starts below.]

The chest x-ray is normal; the pelvic film shows fractures on the right side of both anterior and posterior rami as well as a 2-cm displacement of the right sacroiliac joint.

It depends at this point on how the patient feels, whether her physical exam has changed [ ] at all, and whether her vital signs have changed or stabilized. At this point, it's probably wise to get another hematocrit to see if she needs to go to the OR.

You didn't mention it before, but she probably has MAST trousers on her. Start O-negative blood and put her in the ICU with an attempt to resuscitate her. Assuming these were the only injuries that we found in the rest of survey and that her hematocrit continues to drop while she is stable hemodynamically, I would consider angiography. Otherwise, I would consider alternatives such as pelvic fixation vs. operative management. [3]

Displacement on the right? Well, the first step is to try to ascertain a little more **field information about the direction of impact.** We've learned that impact is one of the more important factors to guide therapy with pelvic fractures. The geography of the fractures as seen on the plain film may be misleading. On the one hand, the fracture may look fairly innocuous, even if there is significant unhinging in the posterior elements. On the other hand, considerable displacement from lateral impact may involve little threat of immediate bleeding. Any more information? Is this a head-on collision or a lateral collision?

[The Attending's think-aloud continues.]

There was no information about the direction of impact.

The second step, after asking about the force of impact, is to look at the **geography of the fracture** for evidence of where the injury is and **how much displacement has occurred.** Of course, the **posterior elements are far more commonly associated with significant hemorrhage**, and greater displacement—particularly if it is **vertical**—would suggest shearing of the internal epigastric arterial arcade with associated injury. You described a 2-cm vertical displacement of the sacroiliac. Regardless of the lack of confirmation from the field about impact, this injury would be **deemed at high-risk for pelvic hemorrhage.**

The woman with this type of impact who arrives with a pulse of 130 (I use 120 as a cutoff) should be **assumed to have ongoing hypovolemic shock from the onset.** The mindset ought to be to look for occult bleeding. The onus is on you to disprove ongoing active torso hemorrhage. You have already addressed this important issue—you have looked at the chest, and the pelvis suggests a problem, but you haven't excluded the abdomen. Because the patient has no open fractures, you don't have to worry about other sources.

First, we're assuming ongoing hemorrhage. Now we are down to the question of whether the source is the abdomen, the pelvis, or both. Right now we can assume that the pelvis is at least a major contributor, but we're not certain that it is the primary focus.

My intuition would be, first, to secure the ABCs (airways, breathing, and circulation) ④—to get the patient resuscitated. And once you begin that, then the next step is to sort out whether the pelvis or abdomen is the source of hemorrhage.

Twenty minutes after arrival the patient's BP is 80/palp, her pulse is 160, she has two cutdowns going wide open with lactated Ringer's. A semi-open, supraumbilical DPL has been done that shows 300,000 red blood cells per high-power field.

The vital signs confirm the concern about active hemorrhage. And **the DPL is a pivotal tool for early triage to separate the bleeding in the abdomen and the pelvis.** If the DPL has been done with good technique and the return of fluid is good—i.e., 750 cc of 1,000 cc—you have a **very powerful adjunct ⑤ as to where you move now.** If you have confidence in the DPL, 300,000 red cells suggest that in fact the peritoneal cavity is not the major source of ongoing bleeding. Therefore your attention should be directed to the pelvis.

If you believe that the pelvis is a major source of bleeding, both the orthopedic service and the radiologist should be contacted as early as possible. The data you have now offer persuasive evidence that you are dealing with a major threat of bleeding from the pelvis. This hypothesis is further strengthened by the absence of rib fractures or other evidence of upper torso injuries, such as clavicular fractures or head injury. This suggests that the major impact was to the pelvic region, probably a frontal impact with opening up of the pelvis.

What would be your next therapeutic move?

Now the big **fork in the decision tree is angiography or skeletal fixation.** That decision is predicated on (1) the patient's physiologic response to resuscitation, (2) the geography of the fractures and the assurance from the orthopedic service that skeletal fixation will in fact have an impact, and (3) the resources within your institution. The problem in this particular patient is an extremely disruptive posterior component fracture. I assume she has anterior fragments as well— essentially a Malgaigne type fracture with vertical displacement. Although the external skeletal fixture may have some salutary effect, it probably is not going to be as definitive. So unless other fractures come into play and convince you otherwise, at this particular juncture, with this magnitude of hemorrhage, the inclination is to **move on to pelvic angiography,** recognizing that of all such fractures you see, pelvic angiography is warranted in less than 5%. All the contributing factors suggest that you're dealing with that really unusual situation.

The patient is taken to the angiography suite. An angiogram identifies no active extravasation of dye. By this time she has had 4 units of blood, her hematocrit is 22, her systolic BP is 100, and her pulse rate is 140.

First of all, she clearly needs to be resuscitated, with careful attention to coagulation problems. And then she should be taken to the OR for skeletal fixation. Preliminary to skeletal fixation, or concurrent with it, **a repeat DPL should be done to make absolutely certain that we are not dealing with ongoing intraabdominal bleeding.**

In the OR the external fixator is placed. We're now 3 hours from the time she hit the ED. A repeat DPL is grossly positive.

How has she responded to resuscitation? How much blood has she had?

She has had 6 units by now. Her crit remains about 25, her pressure is in the 100–110 range, and her pulse is 120–130.

Of course, the natural tendency is to assume that the grossly positive DPL is falsely positive because of extravasation out of the pelvis from the fractures. Unfortunately, in this situation of virtually **refractory shock, I don't think you can afford to make that assumption.** Therefore, before she is taken out of the OR, I would perform a **laparotomy.** [6] I would say that concurrently she needs the Swan-Ganz catheter and the full-bore resuscitation mode. But she also needs a laparotomy, and this is the time to do it.

At laparotomy, a small grade 1 laceration of the spleen is found. Approximately 300 cc of blood is found intraperitoneally. It is easily managed, and there is an enormous hematoma rising out of the pelvis.

Now is the time to ask the angiography staff how confident they are that their angiogram was complete and whether there is a remote possibility of operative impact. If the angiogram was systematic and they had canvassed the potential areas of bleeding, to open the pelvic hematoma would be disastrous. The only recourse you have at this time is to place packs in the pelvis and abdomen with the idea of returning to remove them 24 hours after the hematoma has stabilized.

On review of the arteriographic films in your mind and in the OR, it's clear that they do not entirely exclude extravasation in the pelvis because of technical difficulty.

Assuming you have a reasonably adept interventional radiologist who has done his or her best to curtail the bleeding, at this juncture I still would pack and towel-clip the abdomen. The difference now is that instead of going into the intensive care unit, I would spend the next **hour in the OR resuscitating the patient** and retesting whether in fact we can achieve tamponade in the pelvis.

An hour later the pulse is 160, and the systolic pressure is 100. The patient has received 12 units of blood, and the abdomen is very tense, straining at the towel clips. You are in the OR.

Now we are talking about the 1 in a 1,000 case. We have gone from 5% to .1%. At this juncture you have two choices: to return to angiography and give the radiologists another shot or to intervene yourself in the OR. Unless the radiologists convince me that there will be something magical about their second attempt, I would open the hematoma, isolate the internal hypogastric artery, embolize it with a coagulant slurry on both sides, and ligate the side on which the displaced fracture has occurred. ⑦

Resident: You said the original DPL was 300,000. How come you didn't do a laparotomy? With a mashed pelvis, you're not going to do a laparotomy unless you pull 10 cc of gross blood?

Attending: That's right. But that concept is not widely recognized. Our paper in 1986 is the first to distinguish the specific role of grossly positive aspirate. We didn't emphasize it in that paper because we thought it was sort of intuitive. But since that paper many people have told us that it was the first time they recognized the concept. This is when you use DPL. Frankly I think DPL got its bad name because we operated on the basis of conventional criteria (i.e., >100,000 RBCs/hpf). We opened up a bunch of patients with 100,000–300,000 red cells and found a really rinky-dink spleen injury. By then there is a huge hematoma, the patient has coagulopathy, and by the time you get down to angiography, you've lost that window of opportunity. And hypothetically, if you read the recent case report in the *New England Journal* and the similar recent expanded editorial in *Surgery*, I couldn't disagree more. In a situation almost identical to this, it is recommended to go to the OR and do a laparotomy. And that's the last place you want to be with the patient with a bleeding pelvic fracture.

Surgical Observations

1st-Year Resident

① Whereas in other protocols the resident has relied on laboratory tests and x-rays, in this patient the resident decides to rely on "how the patient feels" and her physical exam, both of which in this trauma scenario are *highly unreliable*.

3rd-Year Resident

② The third-year resident has developed three heuristic principles: large-bore axis → early DPL; grossly positive → to OR; and pelvic fractures → treat conservatively. This technique is not seen in the first-year resident's thoughts.

③ At this point the third-year resident decides to use serial hematocrits (appropriate) and, in view of the emphasis on the pelvic fracture heuristic principle, which takes him down a different path from simple intraperitoneal bleeding. This approach stands him in good stead by giving him other thoughts about how to manage the patient with the pelvic fracture, such as pelvic fixation, angiography, and so forth.

Attending Surgeon

④ At this time the attending begins the ABCs, which would be the standard sort of ED algorithm. Before he goes into the rote basic resuscitation, he gets his mind clear on what the *processes* are likely to be.

⑤ In talking about DPL, the surgeon adds the qualifying term "very powerful adjunct," thus giving his version of its specificity and power. He singles it out of all the other data, such as vital signs, hematocrits, and laboratory data, to

(Continued on following page.)

note that it is "very powerful." But he also notes the two or three possibilities that would decrease its power—poor return, no fluid return, and so forth.

[6] Note the multiple factors (rather than one limb of a decision tree) that lead to the laparotomy. Of particular importance is the fact that the patient has refractory shock, even though the surgeon talks about the possibility of ignoring the grossly positive lavage. He is weighing multiple factors that the less experienced surgeon would not weigh but simply acts on reflexively.

[7] It has been very difficult to get this surgeon to open a traumatic pelvic hematoma.

The expert's script has more detailed knowledge and more structure.

Cognitive Psychologist's Commentary: Pelvic Fracture

Remarkable in this think-aloud is the vast difference between the attending and the residents in the amount of detail in what they say. The paper-patient format allows the surgeons to fill in the details according to the possibilities they recognize in the situation.[1] The attending knows a great deal and thus has a lot to fill in.

The paper patient also offers the attending an opportunity to teach. But this is not just idle teaching, for everything he covers is pertinent to the problems with which he is wrestling for this particular patient.

The thoughts of the first-year resident are vague. The resident seems to know nothing about pelvic fracture in particular and instead uses a generic trauma script: "If the patient's vital signs indicate she is in bad shape, take her to the OR, open her up, find out what it is, and take care of it."

The third-year resident has the basic script for pelvic fracture: treat conservatively. The script includes the conflict between pelvic and abdominal bleeding, as expressed in his attention to grossly positive DPL.

The attending surgeon knows a large amount of information about pelvic fracture in particular. He lays out the distinctions one can make: specifically, the different types of pelvic bone displacement that are likely in accidents involving different mechanisms and their implications for hemorrhage. For example, vertical displacement of posterior elements suggests shearing of the internal iliac arterial arcade. His script leads him to assume hemorrhage and to focus on figuring out its source, in this case, pelvic versus abdominal (or both).

So far we have summarized the attending surgeon's more detailed response to the same basic information that the residents received. What he says later goes further than the residents because the presenter gave him additional information, pushing the interstices of his script and not letting the situation resolve into any particular category. As the attending surgeon noted, soon they were talking about the 1 in 1000 case. And that is the point: with sufficient experience and thought, one's knowledge—one's collection of scripts—is sufficiently differentiated that it can deal with even the very rare case.

---

1. Abernathy CM, Hamm RM: Surgical Intuition. Philadelphia, PA, Hanley & Belfus, 1994, chapter 4.

42. RECTAL BLEEDING

A 62-year-old man who passed bright red blood per rectum just that afternoon presents in the ED. He has had no prior symptoms, his vital signs are stable, and he looks pretty good. What are your thoughts on what it might be? How you might work it up?

3rd-Year Resident

I want to make sure he is not currently in a dangerous situation. The vital signs are very important, and I want to proceed with the physical examination and rule out the problems that would be a major threat at this point. I don't check the hematocrit because he is bleeding per rectum. The greatest danger is that he could be bleeding large amounts that may get him into trouble shortly.

His hematocrit is 30, his vital signs are stable, and he looks healthy.

From that point, in terms of diagnosis, the most important thing I am going to look for is colon cancer in this age group. Other possibilities include diverticular disease, hemorrhoids, vascular malformations, and so forth. The vascular malformations are a bit less common. Also, in terms of his work-up, I will be thinking therapeutically. But in this case, therapy will depend highly on what we find in the work-up. I want to listen to his lungs and check his heart. The abdominal exam and the rectal exam, of course, are going to be very important.

Chief Resident

In that age range, you worry about everyday run-of-the-mill problems, such as hemorrhoids. You would also be worried about things for which he is at risk, such as colon cancer and other tumors of the bowel that could cause bleeding.

For the work-up, **first I would scope him from below.** I would do a history and physical examination to find out if he has any significant risk factors. Then I would see if he has any previous history of hemorrhoids, symptoms associated with something more significant, such as weight loss, and so forth. Finally, after doing a physical examination, including a rectal examination, I would probably do a sigmoidoscopy myself.

On sigmoidoscopy, you see nothing but bright red blood and stool. You don't see any hemorrhoids, and you don't feel any on the rectal lining. But you see blood that is bright red.

At that point I would want his laboratory examination.

His crit is 30.

Attending Surgeon

A 62-year-old man with bright red rectal bleeding in the ED—I would assess for shock, do a physical exam, type, and cross him. On rectal exam, I can't feel anything, but I may use an anoscope at the time to rule out hemorrhoids. I may insert an NG tube into his stomach and aspirate to see if there is any blood, realizing that, because 15% of upper GI lesions won't show in the aspirate, I could still be missing it. After that, if the bleeding is significant, I would proceed probably with a **tagged red-cell scan.** They're not often definitive, but I would say that in half the cases I get some sort of information about whether the problem is in the right colon or left colon. It won't tell me what the problem is.

Then I may think about trying colonoscopy. In fact, I would try. Sometimes

On the rectal exam you see bright red blood. The abdominal exam is normal.

With a hematocrit of 30 and knowledge of where the bleeding started, the patient may have bright red blood from a massive bleed high in the GI tract. More commonly, bright red blood comes from lower GI bleeding. You say the rectal exam is normal as well?

Just blood on the examining finger—bright red blood. On the ward he pours out about a liter and a half of bright red blood, and the nurse calls you. His blood pressure is down to 60, and you decide you have got to go to the OR. You open him up, and in his colon you see dark blood. You can see through the serosa from the cecum all the way around to the distal sigmoid colon.

First, before we go into the OR, we haven't given any blood—and if he's bleeding. . . .

We're going to give him some blood.

And if he is bleeding that rapidly, I want to identify the site of the bleeding before going to the OR.

What do you mean?

If he is bleeding a liter and a half a short period after he's admitted to the floor, then you could do a selective arteriogram or a tagged cell study—nuclear medicine study. He is bleeding fast enough at that point to identify a site of bleeding in the GI tract.

It's low but acceptable. I would colonoscope him from below. You can have an upper GI bleed that is significant and manifests itself as bright red blood in the passage, if it's vast enough to come out. However, given the fact that he's relatively asymptomatic and stable, that's fairly unlikely. An upper GI bleed is a possibility, but I start off looking at his lower GI tract first.

You try to colonoscope him, but there is so much blood and so much stool that you just can't get the scope beyond where you were with the sigmoidoscope.

Is active bleeding coming out? Or just blood-stained matter?

There is red blood in the colon.

There are several other techniques to evaluate the area when you can't determine by visualization whether or not it's bleeding. You can do a bleeding scan, or you can do arteriography for ongoing bleeding. Each of those requires approximately 0.5–1.0 cc of blood production per minute to be able to visualize.

You do the red-cell scan, and it looks to you like the tagged red cells are diffused throughout the whole colon. No one single spot stands out. The nurse in the ICU reports that he has just passed about a liter and a half of bright red blood. You decide to go to the OR. The colon is full of blood from the cecum around to the distal sigmoid colon.

Without any obvious source of bleeding, I probably would be tempted to do a left colectomy and take the chance that it would stem the site of the bleeding.

there is so much blood and so much junk—feces and what not—that you have to be very persistent. But sometimes you can move the colonoscope around, and if you can, **sometimes you can see an area of fresh blood on the mucosa, which lets you know the general area that you need.** That's one of the most important things—not the diagnosis, but the general area.

We do the colonoscopy—maybe we get the information, maybe we don't. The patient has massive bleeding, which is typical of angiodysplasia—by the way, I have that in my mind. If we go to the OR, and the colon is absolutely full of blood, I've got some information if I saw the sigmoid diverticula with a bright red thing on colonoscopy. If I have no information at all, it's really trouble.

You can try **segmental clamping** if he is actively bleeding and see if the blood increases between the clamps. You can actually try—and this is really tough—to scope him at the time, but the rigid scope usually gets contaminated with all the blood and feces. **With a liter and a half of blood out in the bed, if I am absolutely down against the wall, I take out all his colon.**

Further Observations from the Attending Surgeon

You've got to know the hardness of your data. A tagged red-cell scan is a "dotagram"—maybe the dots are in the central abdomen, maybe they're a little on the right side. You don't just say, "Oh, it's in the right colon." Then the patient loses a liter and a half of blood from his rectum and you take out his right colon. But the bleeding was from the redundant sigmoid, even though it appeared in the right abdomen. When critical decisions come up, you have to be critical, too.

But if I had a good enough hint, if I had scoped him and seen this sort of staining of bright blood between the stool and stuff, then I may try to take out the left or right colon, the transverse colon—the whatever colon—to feel for polyps, to feel for cancer, to do all that. But if you can't figure it out, you have to be heavy-duty.

This case shows the more definite need for intuition, as opposed to the think-aloud protocols that are simply reflections of the algorithm. For these scenarios, on the other hand, it is very unlikely that algorithms will ever be written. The decisions and thoughts have characteristics of an algorithmic mode, but ultimately they involve more the intuitive type of thought process.

A nonyielding search pushes the script to the limit.

Cognitive Psychologist's Commentary: Rectal Bleeding

The surgeons' responses to the problem posed by the patient with rectal bleeding illustrate what people have to do to solve diagnostic problems—they have to *search*.[1,2] Responding appropriately to rectal bleeding depends on finding the cause—where it is bleeding and why. And *where* is the more important consideration at the outset. The surgeons have a mental representation of the possibilities and sequentially try each one to evaluate whether it is correct. In this case they must search through the possible locations of the source of bleeding, using various procedures to determine the actual source: sigmoidoscope, colonoscope, abdominal palpation, and x-ray visualization with radioisotope-tagged red blood cells. Any of these procedures may potentially yield a find, but the presenter frustrates the surgeons' search to increase the value of the exercise. When surgeons know how to conduct the search, their knowledge, as we have demonstrated throughout this book, is contained in a script that makes it easily accessible. As the presenter frustrates the first responses that such scripts provide, the surgeons' scripts are pushed to their limits and tested.

The word "search" is not just a convenient metaphor for describing problem solving. When researchers in artificial intelligence set out to program computers to solve problems, a formalized search procedure turned out to be an essential part of the problem-solving process.[3] And this metaphor in turn is the basis of our understanding of how people solve certain types of problems.[1,4]

A basic assumption of the theory that problem solving requires search is that people can think of a relatively large set of possible "states of the world"—things that may be true.

With this patient, for example, the possible states may include each distinct cause and location of rectal bleeding, as well as the possible evidence associated with each. Some of these states can be reached easily from one's present state (i.e., what one knows now). For example, one can palpate the abdomen or inspect the bed clothes. Reaching other states may require taking steps to intermediate states first, expensive effort (e.g., the tagged blood cell procedure), or personal displeasure (e.g., colonoscopy in a bloody unprepared colon).

Search is accomplished by moving from state to state. An important distinction can be made between search that is strictly internal (i.e., it moves from state to state in a mental representation of the situation without actually doing anything) and search that is external (i.e., it involves looking in the world and actually produces new information). In the internal mental search, one imagines what information would be gained if one moved to a certain state and what one could do with the information. On this basis one decides to which state to move (or to which sequence of states, sketching out a path). Internal search uses evidence that is already at hand but has not, until now, been put together.

The person who is searching "in the world" to solve a problem picks a state and moves to it, for example, by performing a procedure and observing the information it produces. When one tests a possibility, such as whether the source of the blood is in the sigmoid colon, one is looking for "yes, it is right" or "no, it is wrong." But one can also learn other information that may force a change in the representation of the whole problem. New information may change the list of possible states and force one to rethink the search strategy before deciding to which state to move next.

Medical problem solving involves a combination of real search and mental search, in which the mental search scouts ahead, solving by internal search the problem of which move to make next in the external search. By this procedure, one moves through the possible states, from one to another, aiming to arrive at a state in which the problem is solved. In both humans and computers, success often depends on being able to remember where one has been so one can backtrack after awhile if a path does not seem to be leading toward the goal.

The surgeons' case is a dynamic rather than a static problem. Changes can take place independently of what the surgeon does in his or her search—the patient can bleed in his bed, or there may be a sudden onset of abdominal pain. Furthermore, the problem is an uncertain situation. The surgeon may check out a possibility and get misleading information. Consequently, even in the external search it may be necessary to backtrack, to keep something in mind as a possibility even if the standard check found no evidence for it. One must be ready in one's search to come back and revisit an earlier state.

In the case of rectal bleeding, as with many other surgical problems, the external search focuses on *location* rather than *cause*. Once the location is found, finding the cause should be easy—and the cause may make no difference in the immediate treatment (e.g., a bleeding portion of colon would be resected, no matter what the cause). However, the search through possible causes (e.g., hemorrhoids, cancer, angiodysplasia) should not be neglected, because possible causes may suggest other evidence to look for or other locations to check.

How is the surgeon's use of search to solve problems integrated with surgical scripts? Surgeons acquire a script through experience with a particular type of patient problem, and only knowledge and skills that are actually used are included in the script. A script for hemorrhoids may not include knowledge about how to handle the problem the paper patient presents—how to find the source of rectal bleeding—because it presumes the source is known. Rectal bleeding, as presented in this think-aloud, falls between the territories covered by most surgical scripts. The needed knowledge may best be organized in a separate script for rectal bleeding itself. Most textbooks do not present information organized to be pertinent to the problem of rectal bleeding; thus residents have to learn the scripts from exposure to cases or from reading think-alouds such as this one.[3]

Everyone faces situations in which they have to search for a solution outside the areas for which they have well-developed scripts. The theory that problem solving is like search offers ideas on how to do so.

Learn general search strategies. If you know a general strategy for searching, you can apply it even to a situation in which you have not searched before. However, the general problem-solving strategies are often difficult for residents to access, and hence they may miss solutions that are within their reach.[4] It may take more time and careful thought than a search in a familiar area, but it can be done[5] if you remember to try it.

Get more states in mind to have more to search through. You cannot move to a state in the internal mental search unless that state, that idea, is active in your mind. Ideas are accessible when they are activated by thoughts that already are active.[6] But you can direct the process by what you choose to pay attention to. Therefore, when engaged in a search that has not yet been successful, it may be useful to open your mind, to be sensitive to ideas that appear but may fade unless you pay attention them—for example, by putting them into words. Visual imagery may be useful in thinking about the problem, because an idea may come to mind in the visual mode even though its name did not come to mind in the verbal mode.[7]

Prioritize. You cannot completely explore all the states of which you can think. Do the most important first. "Most important" is a function of how likely the possibility is, how easy to test, how costly if you find nothing, and related considerations.

Keep track. Don't forget to consider a possibility. Don't forget to come back to check out priority number 3 after number 1 and number 2 have failed to yield a solution.

Remember that some information is uncertain. Given that some decisions about the fruitfulness of a certain path are based on unreliable information, don't put out of mind completely a possibility that you have considered and rejected. As new information comes in or other possibilities are eliminated, a rejected possibility may become viable again and worth reexploring.

Several strategies just reviewed—opening one's mind, being sensitive to faint ideas, following a barely perceptible scent—are the kind of mental activity usually associated with pleasant excitement and lack of stress. Yet the surgeon is asked to perform this mental search while engaged in the physical steps of gathering information—in this case, for example, while the surgeon is pushing a scope through blood and feces. People's usual responses to blood and feces are disgust and revulsion—tightening the lips, contracting the nostrils, and holding the breath. Such physical reactions affect the mental attitude as well, for the mind is in the body and participates in its reactions. The closing of the nostrils may bring with it a closing of the mind. This is not just a poetic analogy—steeling oneself, narrowing one's attention so that one can go through with a procedure, no matter how unpleasant, may help one complete the procedure physically but may prevent the thoughts necessary to make full use of the information gained.

What do surgeons need for their mental searches to be effective in unpleasant circumstances? They need *well-learned scripts*, containing search strategies for the particular problem (e.g., rectal bleeding), so that they can carry out the search even though their minds may be a little constricted by the unpleasant situation. They may need a strategy of setting aside time for thinking when they are not feeling disgusted; for example, they may need to avoid decisions until they have cleaned up.

And they may need professional behavior from the support staff. Observers blowing off steam in reaction to blood and feces may distract the surgeon's attention from the necessary mental search. The surgeon himself or herself may need to express disgust or to joke and laugh about it. But staff who have no thinking responsibilities in the situation shouldn't let their reactions interfere with the thinking of surgeons who do have such responsibilities.

Like most people, doctors in training are polite and tend not to think or to talk about feces. This social habit may cause them not to do much mental practice of their search strategies for rectal bleeding. Because of this neglect, their script for rectal bleeding may develop slowly, lagging behind their scripts for other cases (an instance of "case specificity"[8]). To counter this tendency, their teachers sometimes need to hold their noses to it, to make them observe cases, or to lead them in problem-solving exercises. It is hoped that surgical think-alouds such as this can make it easier and more pleasant for residents to acquire the scripts and search strategies they need to be effective at searching, for example, for the causes of rectal bleeding.

1. Abernathy CM, Hamm RM: Surgical Intuition. Philadelphia, PA, Hanley & Belfus, 1994, chapter 5.
2. Abernathy CM, Hamm RM: Surgical Intuition. Philadelphia, PA, Hanley & Belfus, 1994, chapter 9.
3. Rich E: Artifical Intelligence. New York, McGraw-Hill, 1983.
4. Abernathy CM, Hamm RM: Surgical Intuition. Philadelphia, PA, Hanley & Belfus, 1994, chapter 11.
5. Perkins DN, Salomon G: Are cognitive skills context-bound? Educ Res 18(1):16–25, 1989.
6. Abernathy CM, Hamm RM: Surgical Intuition. Philadelphia, PA, Hanley & Belfus, 1994, chapter 3.
7. Abernathy CM, Hamm RM: Surgical Intuition. Philadelphia, PA, Hanley & Belfus, 1994, chapter 10.
8. Elstein AS, Shulman LS, Sprafka SA: Medical problem solving: A ten-year retrospective. Eval Health Prof 13:5–36, 1990.

43. ACUTE PAIN IN LEG

A 73-year-old man is referred to you with acute onset of pain in the left leg 6 hours previously. He now has no pedal pulses by Doppler ultrasonic flowmeter. He has no known cardiac problem and is in normal sinus rhythm. What are your thoughts? What would you do?

2nd-Year Resident

This is an acute-onset problem that the patient never had before? The patient has no cardiac problem. My initial concern—with new onset of pain in the leg and no pulses—is the possibility of an embolism. The question is where or when.

I would ask him about the five Ps. [1] He does have pain. I would examine him for pallor, paresthesia, and—because he is pulseless in his distal extremities—for hypothermia of his leg. Is his pain out of proportion to the physical findings? That is what I would be concerned about.

I would also get a little more of his history. I know he is an elderly man. Does he have any evidence of peripheral vascular disease or any history of prior surgery, abdominal aneurysm, carotid disease—anything that would indicate atherosclerotic disease? Does he have a history of atrial fibrillation. [2] Such information would also give me a possible etiology for the pain in his legs. Maybe I can look back in his chart. Does he have a history of pulse deficit to begin with? Are the pedal pulses now palpable? Is this a new finding? I think all of that information is important. I would do a course of vascular examination to see if he has other pulses. I would listen to his heart and lungs and see if there are any bruits anywhere. [3]

Chief Resident

My thoughts are that an acute process in the man's left leg has caused him to lose his pulses, and I assume that no pulses are detectable by Doppler. So he has absolutely no pulses below the groin. My feeling is that you have to rule out acute occlusion versus embolism, **thrombosis versus embolism.**

All my energies would be directed initially toward establishing a history and finding out whether he ever had any evidence of cardiac arrhythmias or is predisposed to an embolus. If I could ascertain that the findings are consistent with embolus, I would take him immediately to the operating room for an embolectomy. If I could not make that determination and if diagnosis was acute thrombosis, then I would have to do other procedures, such as arteriography. [4]

Attending Surgeon

My thought is that he has either an embolism or thrombosis of the left lower extremity, and we need to evaluate him. I would get a history and a physical exam. I would check his pulses to see if they are palpable. I would see if he has any Doppler signals in his legs. If not, then I would do an arteriogram. [6]

You decide to do an arteriogram, which shows a completely occluded left superficial femoral artery with no visualization of the trifurcation. The profunda femoris is open, and the aorta iliac vessels are nicely open. What now?

Since the trifurcation is occluded, my concern is an acute process. I would consider taking him to the operating room. I am not as much concerned about left superficial femoral artery occlusion if the patient has no history of claudication. If there appears to be no collateral circulation, I have to assume that this is an acute process. I would take the patient to the operating room and do a thrombectomy.

Are there any alternatives?

There sure are. It is 6 hours out, but some studies indicate that you can give streptokinase or urokinase. First I would put the patient on heparin and see. In an acute situation— under 6 hours—you have a chance to save the leg. I think you need to take the patient to the operating room and do an embolectomy.

The contralateral leg is normal? Everything is open in the contralateral leg? At this point the problem is outflow, and if the leg is frankly cadaveric, time is critical. Is there any muscle loss? Do I have time to try systemic therapy in an attempt to open up both vessels to see what the underlying anatomy was before this occlusion?

The leg appears severely ischemic.

At this point I see only one basic choice: to take the patient to the operating room, open up the groin at the left femoral artery, and do a thrombectomy as best I can on the operating room table. And I would probably instill **intraoperative urokinase** while I am calling for x-ray to shoot an arteriogram on the operating table. I want to see if I can get any vessels in the lower leg opened for outflow. [5]

Is there any reconstitution of the lower vessels? [7]

No visualization of the trifurcation.

I would go to the operating room and do a femoral thrombectomy.

How would you do that?

I would cut down on his left femoral artery, isolate the vessels, open up the common femoral, and put a Fogarty catheter down the superficial femoral artery.

At the finish of the procedure, you have no pedal pulses by Doppler.

I do an arteriogram to see what shows after I have done the thrombectomy.

The operative arteriogram reveals that the trifurcation is now open and the anterior tibial artery is opened half way down the leg. That is the only outflow.

In the operating room, I would probably give him urokinase.

You still have no palpable pulses in the foot. I assume you mean a bolus?

At this point I would still like to salvage his leg. I would leave the catheter in place and try to drip in the urokinase. Then I would bring him back to the ICU, watch him, and, depending on what happened, make new decisions as we went along.

Surgical Observations

2rd-Year Resident

[1] The resident obviously wants more or better hints from the history. But his questions (such as the 5 P's) are unlikely to lead to the correct diagnosis or therapy. Instead they are "descriptive" (like the body of a radiology report). Questions about the signs and symptoms of ischemia are of no help in figuring out the etiology of the ischemia, which may determine therapy.

[2] First the resident asked about "heart disease," but a few sentences later he is more focused, asking specifically about atrial fibrillation.

[3] The resident offers no plan for the diagnostic work-up beyond the history and physical exam. In fact, there is no speculation on where this case may lead in terms of therapeutic options.

Chief Resident

[4] The chief resident nicely identifies the embolus vs. thrombosis differential in the preexisting disease problem, but he is a little slower than the attending at realizing that almost certainly the next step is an arteriogram.

[5] A nice plan is formulated, including not only "going to the operating room," but also what is likely to transpire there. The resident has a solid, complete surgical script.

Attending Surgeon

[6] The attending surgeon rapidly defines the problem and sketches a plan of attack. This is a good surgical script with little waffling or extraneous material.

[7] Once the rather sketchy verbal findings of the arteriogram are revealed, the attending surgeon has only one question; is there any reconstitution of the lower vessels? He focuses on this as the single important fact, along with the decision to operate.

Expert scripts support expert judgments.

Cognitive Psychologist's Commentary:
Acute Pain in Leg

The thoughts of the second-year resident contrast starkly with those of the chief resident and the attending surgeon. The novice has a great deal of knowledge, but it is not organized for effective response to the patient. In terms of Anderson's analysis[1,2] of cognitive skill, the second-year resident seems to be relying on "declarative" knowledge here, whereas the others are using "procedural" knowledge.[3,4]

Declarative knowledge is knowledge of what is, whereas procedural knowledge focuses on method or "how to." Declarative knowledge is stored in memory as sentences—facts stated in words. Examples include: "If a patient has thrombosis, you can use streptokinase or urokinase," or "signs of embolism in the lower extremities include pallor, paresthesia." Procedural knowledge, in contrast, governs people's responses to situations, but the responses do not depend on interpreting the meaning of words. For example, the attending's response to the initial description is a plan that came to mind as the result of a single recognition: "This is embolism or thrombosis, and my plan for dealing with them is as follows." If not required to say it aloud, the surgeon simply would have done it; he does not need to recall sentences, to think about their meaning, to deduce implications, and so forth.

It is evident from the amount of what the second-year resident has to say that he has a great deal of relevant knowledge. When he recognizes the possibility of an embolism, for example, he recalls the five Ps acronym and steps part way through it. He knows that old men's leg arteries can have emboli or thromboses, and he knows that you can find information in their histories about conditions that may cause either or both. But his knowledge is not as complete as that of the more experienced surgeons, and it is not organized for use in this context. The other two immediately structure their thinking about the patient in terms of embolus versus thrombosis; their thoughts go to signs that may help them to differentiate the two rather than to signs that are associated with both.[5] The second-year resident knows both concepts but does not organize his thoughts around the contrast between them. The experienced surgeons' scripts quickly lead them to recognize that arteriography is required (the attending surgeon is a little quicker than the chief resident), whereas the second-year resident does not mention it.

One key distinction between the second-year resident, with his undirected search through his knowledge, and the more experienced surgeons, with their scripted responses, is **their sense of what is important.** The inexperienced resident is not well focused. He seems not to have thought about where he will take a given line of reasoning—to which diagnostic or treatment decisions it will lead. This is not to say that he does not differentiate between facts on the basis of their importance. He states explicitly that the list of possible symptoms for which he would look in the chart includes information that is "very important." But his sense of importance is diffuse: facts are important if they are associated with any of the diseases in question.

The experienced physicians, in contrast, have a much more specific conception of which factors are crucial at each point, and this conception provides them with a different basis for judging what information is important and what decisions must be made. For example, the chief resident expresses a sense of urgency at the outset: "All my energies would be directed initially toward . . . finding out whether he ever had any evidence of cardiac arrhythmia or is predisposed to an embolus." He knows he has to respond quickly to an embolus. The sense of importance that motivates the chief resident's responses comes from (1) having the script and (2) having had the responsibility for caring for this sort of patient.

After the results of the arteriogram, another difference between the novice and experienced surgeons appears. The experienced surgeons address their attention to the factors that would make them choose to operate. For example, the chief resident focuses on the condition of the leg—is it dying? When the presenter answers yes, the chief resident is off to the operating room. The experts are secure in their judgments about the seriousness of the situation. The second-year resident, on the other hand, can be talked out of his decision to operate just by being asked whether there are any alternatives. This can happen, in part, because he has not requested from the presenter the information that he needs to drive his decision; he does not yet know what that would be.

The second-year resident knows the functional roles of all the elements of the situation: the ways the vessels can become blocked, the ways to unblock them, the ongoing damage to the ischemic limb, the effects of anticoagulating drugs. But he does not know how to combine these factors into a big picture and hence does not know how to make judgments of danger, of urgency, or of the appropriateness of a treatment based on this knowledge.[6] We can expect that as he continues learning, he will acquire first the scripts with the appropriate plans and later the judgment that enables him to use the scripts flexibly.

---

1. Anderson JR: The Architecture of Cognition. Cambridge, MA, Harvard University Press, 1983.
2. Anderson JR: Cognitive Psychology and its Implications, 3rd ed. New York, W.H. Freeman and Co., 1990.
3. Lesgold A: Problem solving. In Sternberg RJ, Smith EE (eds): The Psychology of Human Thought. New York, Cambridge University Press, 1988, pp 188–213.
4. Abernathy CM, Hamm RM: Surgical Intuition. Philadelphia, PA, Hanley & Belfus, 1994, chapter 4.
5. Abernathy CM, Hamm RM: Surgical Intuition. Philadelphia, PA, Hanley & Belfus, 1994, chapter 6.
6. Abernathy CM, Hamm RM: Surgical Intuition. Philadelphia, PA, Hanley & Belfus, 1994, chapter 8.

INDEX

Page numbers in **boldface type** indicate individual think-alouds.

Abdominal aortic aneurysm, **162–165**
Abdominal sepsis vs. pulmonary sepsis, 139
Action, expert's knowledge organized for, 167–169
  recognition and, in experts' rules, 72
"Action" hypotheses, of expert surgeons, 51–53
Adenocarcinoma, of rectum, **95–101**
  of stomach, **63–65**
Adenoma, villous, of rectum, **93–94**
Adjustment probability, 12
"Aha" phenomenon, 126
Algorithms, skipping, 13–14
  versus master surgeon, 69–70
Ambiguity, handling of, by master surgeon, 90–92
Analysis, in timing of operation, 119–120
Anatomy, patient's, visualization by experts vs. novices, 172–173
Anchoring and adjustment, concept of, in assessment of operative risk, 11–14
Appendicitis, intuitive judgment in, **85–87**
Arteriotomy, technique for, 9

"Big picture," master surgeon's focus on, 78, 111, 127, 143
Billroth procedures, for gastric outlet obstruction, 71–72
Biopsy, of breast mass, decision making in, **35–38**
Bleeding duodenal ulcer, **81–83**
Breast cancer, infiltrating ductal, **27–28, 29–33**
  lymph node dissection for, 24
Breast mass, **23–25, 35–38**
  biopsy for, 35–38
  breast-conserving approach to, 23, 24, 25
  treatment options for, 23–25, 27–28, 29, 31, 35
  vague, **29–33**
Burn, apartment fire, **108–111**
  campfire, **104–107**
"Buying time" to think about a case, 155–157

Campfire burn, **104–107**
Carotid dissection, acute, **112–116**

Carotid endarterectomy, subsequent to stroke, **7–14**
  timing of, factors in, 118–119
Categorical ambiguity, handling of, 90–92
Categories, of patients, fuzzy boundaries of, 27, 28
  patients who don't fit, handling of, 90–92
  recognized, judgment in response to, 150–151
Caution, appropriate use of, 122–123
  as sign of inexperience, 106–107
Cerebral vascular accident, **116–119**
Chemotherapy, adjuvant, for breast cancer, 27, 29, 31
Chest, stab wound to, **39–41**
Cholangiography, for pancreatic mass, 55
Cholecystectomy, laparoscopic, **148–151**
Choledochojejunostomy, Roux-en-Y, 59
Cognitive feedback, in teaching expert judgment, 134
Coloanal anastomosis, technique for, 95–98
Conservative management, inexperience as cause of, 106–107

Decision making, expert. *See* Expert judgments
  knowledge of options in, 82
Decision problems, nature of, 133
Decisions, role of recognition in, 82
  "tough," 21
Declarative knowledge, 188–189
Diagnosis, absence of, irrelevance to decision to operate, 51–52
  differential, creation of, 76, 77–79
Differential diagnosis, creation of, 76, 77–79
Disease frequency, role in disease recognition, 77–79
Duodenal ulcer, bleeding, **81–83**

Endarterectomy, carotid, patching in, 10, 12
  technique for, 9–11
Epigastric pain, 63, 67, 71, 158–161
Expectations, effects on reasoning, 44
Expert judgment
  cognitive feedback in teaching of, 134

Expert judgment *(cont.)*
    difficulty in explaining one's, 132–133
    expert scripts and, 188–190
    how to learn, 134
    "if-then" rules in, 64–65, 72–73
    memory probing in, 134–135
    statistical models in, 133
    tradeoffs in, 134
    "weighted averages" in, 133–134
Expert surgeon. *See* Master surgeon
Expert systems, rule-based, 64–65, 72–73

Failed procedure, expert/novice approach
    to, 127
False negatives, in surgical decision
    making, 69
Flexible script, of master surgeon, 32–33
Football player, unconscious, **15–18**
Forward thinking, by master surgeon,
    46–47, 126, 147

Gastric outlet obstruction, 71–73
    Billroth procedures for, 71–72
Gastric ulcer, **67–70**
    algorithm for, 68
"Get-out-of-trouble" technical tip, 81
Guiding phrase, concept of, 13

Hands, master surgeon thinks with, 101
Hedging, as strategy for buying time, 123
Hemorrhagic pancreatitis, **146–147**
Hypotheses, "action," of expert surgeons,
    51–53
Hypoxia, small bowel obstruction and,
    75–79

If-then rules, in expert judgments, 64–65,
    72–73
Important, sense of what is, as character-
    istic of master surgeon, 189–190
Inexperience. *See also* Novice
    relationship to convervative manage-
        ment, 106–107
Intuition, in timing of operation, 119–120
Intuitive judgment, in appendicitis, **85–87**

Jaundice, pain with, **152–157**
Judgment. *See also* Expert judgment
    in moderating response to recognized
        categories, 150–151
    integration of multiple inputs in,
        133–134
    intuitive, in appendicitis, **85–87**
Judgment-decision box, 37

"Knowing-in-action," concept of, 56–57
Knowledge
    activation of, by master surgeons,
        31–33
    as strength of master surgeon, 62
    declarative vs. procedural, 188–189
    detail content of, in expert vs. novice,
        178–179
    experience-derived, role in learning, 38
    expert. *See also* Expert judgment
        acquisition process of, 114–115
        general-to-specific movement of,
            114–115
        organization of, 4
    from others, role in learning, 38
    "life," of master surgeon, 21
    structure of, in first-year residents,
        160–161
Kocher maneuver, 49

Laparoscopic cholecystectomy, **148–151**
Left lower quadrant pain, **166–169**
Leg, acute pain in, **186–190**
Life knowledge, of master surgeons,
    21
Liver laceration, from motor vehicle
    accident, **140–145**
Liver metastases, **45–47**
Lower quadrant pain, left, **166–169**
    right, **85–87**
Lumpectomy vs. mastectomy, 23–25,
    27–28, 29–33

Marriage of Kakra, 144
Mastectomy, for breast cancer, 23–25,
    27–28, 29–33
    modified radical, technique for, 30
Master surgeon
    "action" hypotheses of, 51–53
    action-oriented knowledge structure of,
        167–169
    anchoring and adjustment of operative
        risk by, 11–14
    "buying time" strategies used by,
        155–157
    certainty as characteristic of decision
        making of, 93–94
    complexity of ideas of, 127
    decision making of, "sureness" as
        characteristic of, 93–94
    degree of caution in thinking of, 123
    experience of, role in decision making,
        25
    explanation by, as teaching tool, 147
    flexibility of scripts of, 32–33

Master surgeon *(cont.)*
  focus on "big picture" by, 78, 111, 127, 143
  focus on control by, 139
  forward thinking by, 46–47, 126, 147
  guiding phrase by, 13
  handling of categorical ambiguity by, 90–92
  intuitive pattern recognition by, 21–22
  "knowing-in-action" by, 56–57
  "knowing what you don't know" facet of, 144
  knowledge of research by, 25
  "life knowledge" of, 21
  mental model of patient constructed by, 138–139
  organization of knowledge by, 4
  ranking of importance of questions by, 145
  recognition of key elements of case by, 17
  recognition of multiple possibilities by, 145
  recognition of scripts by, 31–33
  reliance on specific maxims by, 164–165
  rule-based knowledge of, 64–65, 72–73
  rules of versus thoughts of, 36–38
  search strategies used by, 182–185
  sense of what is important by, 189–190
  short-term memory of, 62
  verbalization of priorities by, 40
  versus algorithm, 69–70
  visualization techniques of, 13, 60, 101, 172–173
Mechanism of injury, in trauma management, 15, 17, 21
Melanoma, **3–5**
Melena, **61–62**
Memory, short-term, of master surgeon, 62
  systematic probing of, in expert judgment, 134–135
Mental models, as mark of expertise, 138–139
Metacognition, in search for better understanding, 144–145
Motor vehicle accident, dilated and sluggish pupils in victim of, **19–22**
  liver laceration from, **140–145**

Novice surgeon
  backward thinking by, 46–47
  conservative management by, 106–107
  reliance on general rules by, 164–165
  reliance on rules of thumb by, 127

Novice surgeon *(cont.)*
  reliance on specific rules by, 110–111
  script learning by, 159–161
  simplicity of ideas of, 127
  use of visualization by, 172–173
Numerical estimation exercise, 13

Operation, risk of, anchoring and adjustment of, 11–14
  timing of, factors involved in, 118–119
  without diagnosis, justification for, 51–52
Options, knowledge of, in good decision making, 82

Pacemaker complication, **124–127**
Pain, acute leg, **186–190**
  epigastric, 63, 67, 71, 158–161
  jaundice with, **152–157**
  left lower quadrant, **166–169**
  right lower quadrant, **85–87**
Pancreas, cancer of, **49–53**
  mass in, **55–57**
Pancreatitis, hemorrhagic, **146–147**
Patch closure, for carotid endarterectomy, 10, 12
Patients, anatomy of, visualization by master surgeon, 13, 60, 101, 172–173
  categories of, fuzzy boundaries of, 27, 28
  mental model of, by master surgeon, 138–139
Pattern recognition, intuitive, by master surgeon, 21–22
Pelvic fracture, **89–92, 174–179**
Physical exam, importance of, to experts vs. novices, 159, 167
Possibilities, multiple, recognition by master surgeon, 145
Postcholecystectomy duct injury, **59–60**
Prejudice, probabilities and, 43–44
Pringle maneuver, 142
Prioritization, in problem solving, 40, 184
Probabilities, knowledge of, in providing perspective for judgment, 150–151
  prejudice and, 43–44
Probability adjustment, 12
Problem solving, search strategies in, 182–185
Procedural knowledge, 188–189
Pruitt-Inahara shunt, technique for insertion of, 9
Pulmonary embolus, 76, 77
Pulmonary nodule, solitary, **128–135**

Pupils, dilated and sluggish, in victim of motor vehicle accident, **19–22**

Reasoning, effect of expectations on, 44
Recognition, as basis for experts' rules, 72
in accessing knowledge, 78–79
in decision making, 82
Rectum, bleeding from, **180–185**
cancer of, **95–101**
villous adenoma of, **93–94**
Residents. *See* Novice surgeon
Retroperitoneal caval injury, 143
Right lower quadrant pain, **85–87**
Roux-en-Y choledochojejunostomy, 59
Rules, as basis of expert systems, 64–65, 72–73
expert knowledge in form of, 72
general versus specific, expert/novice use of, 164–165
specific, reliance of master surgeon on, 164–165
reliance of novice on, 110–111
Rules of thumb, different uses of, 127
in timing of operation, 119–120

Script, surgical. *See* Surgical script
Search, in problem solving, 182–185
strategies for, 184–185
Sepsis, of unknown focus, **136–138**
Small bowel obstruction, **170–173**
hypoxic episode with, **75–79**
Solitary pulmonary nodule, **128–135**
Stab wound to chest, **39–41**
"States of the world," in problem solving, 182–185
Statistical models, in expert judgments, 64–65
Stomach, adenocarcinoma of, **63–65**
Strategies, "buying time," to prolong effective search, 155–157
Stroke, carotid endarterectomy subsequent to, **7–14**
Sureness, in expert surgeon's decision making, 93–94
Surgeon, master. *See* Master surgeon
Surgical scripts, effect of experience and research on, 25

Surgical scripts *(cont.)*
expert, as support for expert judgments, 188–190
expert vs. novice, amount of detail in, 178–179
feedback as method of learning, 160–161
flexible, 32, 33
guiding phrase as core of, 13
recognition of, by master surgeons, 31–33
nonyielding search in, 182–185
solutions outside of, searching for, 184
structure of, in expert vs. novice, 178–179
rigid, 159–161
tactile images in, 56
visual images in, 13, 56, 60, 101, 172–173
visualization in, by experts vs. novices, 172–173

Tactile images, in surgical scripts, 56
Think-alouds, by master surgeons, **3–101**
expert/novice comparisons, **104–190**
Thinking aloud, as preparation for unexpected, 40–41
Thoracic outlet syndrome, **43–44**
Thyroid nodule, **120–123**
"Tough" decisions, 21
Tradeoffs, in learning expert judgment, 134
Trauma, diagnostic patterns in, intuitive recognition by master surgeon, 21–22

Ulcer, duodenal, bleeding, **81–83**
gastric, **67–70**
Unconscious football player, **15–18**

Visual images, in surgical scripts, 13, 56
Visualization, in surgical decision making, 60, 101
master surgeon's use of, 172–173

Weighted averages, in expert judgment, 133–134
Whipple procedure, 152–154
technique of, 49–50

THE SECRETS SERIES®

From Hanley & Belfus, Inc., Philadelphia, Pennsylvania

Charles M. Abernathy, M.D., Series Editor
Professor of Surgery, University of Colorado School of Medicine
Denver, Colorado

The "Secrets" approach has been extraordinarily popular and has given birth to a whole series of books covering . . . Questions You Will Be Asked on Rounds, in the Clinic, in the OR, ED, etc. These mini-textbooks in question/answer format are ideal reviews for examinations, rounds and clinical discussions.

CRITICAL CARE SECRETS
Edited by POLLY E. PARSONS, M.D., Department of Medicine, University of Colorado School of Medicine, Denver, Colorado, and JEANINE P. WIENER-KRONISH, M.D., Department of Anesthesia, University of California, San Francisco, School of Medicine, San Francisco, California • March 1992, 350 pages, illustrated

EMERGENCY MEDICINE SECRETS
Edited by VINCE J. MARKOVCHICK, M.D., PETER T. PONS, M.D., and RICHARD E. WOLFE, M.D., University of Colorado Health Sciences Center, Denver, Colorado • May 1993, 480 pages, illustrated

HEMATOLOGY/ONCOLOGY SECRETS
Edited by MARIE E. WOOD, M.D., and PAUL A. BUNN, Jr., M.D., Department of Medicine, University of Colorado School of Medicine, Denver, Colorado • February 1994, 450 pages, illustrated

MEDICAL SECRETS
Edited by ANTHONY J. ZOLLO, Jr., M.D., Department of Medicine, Baylor College of Medicine, Houston, Texas • June 1991, 574 pages, illustrated

NEUROLOGY SECRETS
Edited by LOREN A. ROLAK, M.D., Department of Neurology, Baylor College of Medicine, Houston, Texas • August 1993, 450 pages, illustrated

OB/GYN SECRETS
Edited by HELEN L. FREDERICKSON, M.D., Saint Joseph Hospital, Denver, Colorado, and LOUISE WILKINS-HAUG, M.D., Ph.D., Brigham and Women's Hospital, Harvard Medical School, Boston, Massachusetts • May 1991, 308 pages, illustrated

PEDIATRIC SECRETS
Edited by RICHARD A. POLIN, M.D., and MARK F. DITMAR, M.D., Department of Pediatrics, University of Pennsylvania School of Medicine and Children's Hospital of Philadelphia, Philadelphia, Pennsylvania • June 1989, 447 pages, illustrated

SPORTS MEDICINE SECRETS
Edited by MORRIS B. MELLION, M.D., Departments of Family Practice and Orthopaedic Surgery (Sports Medicine), University of Nebraska College of Medicine, Omaha, Nebraska • January 1994, 470 pages, illustrated

SURGICAL SECRETS, 2nd edition
Edited by CHARLES M. ABERNATHY, M.D., and ALDEN H. HARKEN, M.D., Department of Surgery, University of Colorado School of Medicine, Denver, Colorado • July 1991, 330 pages, illustrated